OUR HEALTH PLAN

OUR HEALTH PLAN

COMMUNITY GOVERNED HEALTHCARE THAT WORKS

JIM RICKARDS, MD, MBA

NEW YORK

NASHVILLE • MELBOURNE • VANCOUVER

OUR HEALTH PLAN

COMMUNITY GOVERNED HEALTHCARE THAT WORKS

Published in New York, New York, by Morgan James Publishing. Morgan James is a trademark of Morgan James, LLC. www.MorganJamesPublishing.com

The Morgan James Speakers Group can bring authors to your live event. For more information or to book an event visit The Morgan James Speakers Group at www.TheMorganJamesSpeakersGroup.com.

ISBN 9781683502982 paperback
ISBN 9781683503002 eBook
ISBN 9781683502999 hardcover
Library of Congress Control Number: 2016917100

Cover Design by:
Chris Treccani
www.3dogdesign.net

Interior Design by:
Chris Treccani
www.3dogdesign.net

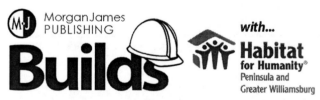

In an effort to support local communities, raise awareness and funds, Morgan James Publishing donates a percentage of all book sales for the life of each book to Habitat for Humanity Peninsula and Greater Williamsburg.

Get involved today! Visit
www.MorganJamesBuilds.com

TABLE OF CONTENTS

INTRODUCTION

As a child, I remember visiting my grandmother in the hospital where she was fighting pneumonia. It was a nice, community hospital, the kind you might find in any number of towns or cities in the U.S. Given her age, she had several chronic medical issues including Parkinson's disease, like the actor Michael J. Fox, which contributed to her current condition. While these issues related to her stay in the hospital, they were just a part of the problem.

She lived alone and could not drive. As a result, she was also probably somewhat depressed. The hospital offered her all the support she needed for the moment, but of course, this came at a cost—not just monetary cost, but the discomfort of being away from home and in an unfamiliar environment.

On this visit, however, she had shown dramatic clinical improvement. I remember my dad kept trying to get answers as to how she would get home, who would help her make appointments with her regular doctors for follow-up, and who was helping transition and coordinate her care.

It turns out, my dad was the one doing most of the work figuring out next steps in the transition of her care. He was a sales manager for an electronics company and, other than the address of the hospital, he didn't really know much about the operations of the healthcare system.

While there was great medical care available and she had incredible providers at the hospital, the building and loosely connected network of providers and services wasn't really a system. There was no group of individuals and entities working together under one common mission and vision, with one global budget, and no way to measure its performance in aggregate.

No, there wasn't a system, but there were many parts of a system working for my grandmother. There were the doctors, of course; the non-emergency medical transportation providers; the insurance company; the meals-on-wheels folks; the pharmacist; and the home health aide, the social worker, and a whole host of others. They were all there to help—but they were doing it in a way that was not coordinated, which resulted in frustration, inefficiency, and probably a lot of waste.

I remember the day came that my grandma was going to be discharged. We went to the hospital early in the morning. My dad asked many questions, trying to figure out next steps.

He traveled a lot for work and knew airlines were, for the most part, able to pull together pilots, mechanics, planes, ticket counter attendants, baggage handlers, etc., all to get individuals where they needed to go with a clear plan detailed on a ticket. They were also able to do this, for the most part, on time and at a cost you clearly knew ahead of traveling.

This didn't seem to be the case when trying to make the short trip from hospital to home. We were finally told by a nurse that the team—in other words, the doctors, the social workers, pharmacists, physical therapists, and transportation service providers—were going to get together to come up with a plan to get Grandma home. We waited and waited. As a kid at the time, I remember I didn't mind the wait because there was cable TV to watch in the room—a real treat in the late 1980s.

Slowly, throughout the course of the day, I realized what was happening. There was no team, there was no meeting, and there was only somewhat of a plan. We had been so naive to think that this system and this team of varied providers worked together and were going to develop a cohesive plan for our grandma recovering from pneumonia.

My grandma was eventually discharged to home and we were able to fumble through the process of helping get her there. But I couldn't help wondering why it had to be this way. I couldn't help comparing the process to my father's at work. Sure, this wasn't air travel, but there were similarities—large, physical structures dedicated to one service, highly skilled professionals, high costs, and the risk of life and death. If we could streamline air travel, why couldn't we do the same with healthcare?

While going through medical school, I kept the idea and possibility of this team, this coordinated effort, in mind. I was always on the lookout for it. I figured that, because my grandmother's facility was a community hospital, they must not have had the resources of the well-funded, tertiary-care academic systems where I received my training. What I learned was that, if anything, these seemingly well-funded systems were even less coordinated, because there were so many more resources, so many more services, and so many more ways to pay and bill for care.

As I began my medical practice in a small town in Oregon, I had fully accepted the healthcare system for what it was, with all its shortcomings in coordinating care. However, my frustration with it continued to grow. As a radiologist—a physician who interprets medical imaging exams such as CAT scans and x-rays—it's not necessarily a good thing to really "get to know" your patients. The exams we perform are expensive and can expose you to radiation, which comes with its own risks. The less frequently we see our patients, sometimes the better, in terms of their health.

What frustrated me was that I was seeing the same patients come back repeatedly: an alcoholic who would have a CAT scan of his brain every Monday because of an *alcohol*-withdrawal seizure, a teenage girl with an unintentional pregnancy for the third time in two years, and a diabetic slowly losing his leg because the disease was poorly controlled.

I knew I was doing everything right interpreting the various imaging exams. My colleagues in internal medicine and the emergency department were delivering great care. The problem is this: ninety-nine percent of patients' lives are lived outside the four walls of a hospital or clinic. Thus, multiple "determinants health"—such as socioeconomic factors, education, and housing—impact them in far greater ways than the medical care they receive.

These determinants, and the those who provide care in these areas, need to be a part of our "healthcare system"—not just our physicians, nurses, and hospitals, but our behavioral health providers, social workers, early childhood learning resources, housing, and transportation providers, as well.

This sounds like a lot, but these are the various aspects of life and community which determine our health. The problem is, these parts don't all work together. They are isolated, fragmented, and don't talk.

This book is the story of how the State of Oregon sought to bring these various pieces together to improve health and reduce costs for the most vulnerable members of the population, patients receiving Medicaid health benefits. This book is for people who may or may not work in a hospital or the medical field and who face the same frustrations my family did while visiting my grandmother.

In this book, you're going to hear about a lot of great ideas and how the power of community turned these ideas into practice to deliver better care and create a true healthcare system. You won't find a lot of technical jargon or references to high-power research. What you will see, though, is how what we've done in Oregon can be accomplished by healthcare professionals and patients everywhere who simply want to develop relationships, work together, and put the control of their healthcare resources back into their communities. This is an approach that worked for us, and I think it can work just about anywhere.

CHAPTER 1:

HEALTHCARE:

THERE IS A BETTER WAY

he issues we face in Yamhill County, Oregon, plus or minus, are the issues that all communities across the country face every day. Healthcare spending is on the rise. Patients and healthcare providers alike are frustrated because they aren't getting great results. Insurance companies are increasing their sway. There is a lack of communication within healthcare provider networks. And, thanks to Obamacare, there is a burgeoning caseload of newly insured patients. We all want and need a better system.

Oregon has decided to address these issues with a new care model for the most economically disadvantaged: the Medicaid population. The approach is the *Coordinated Care Model* and it is delivered through organizations called *coordinated care organizations* or CCOs. This is the story of how one community,

Yamhill County, took healthcare into its own hands and started a CCO. Thus, Yamhill has been able to improve care, lower costs, develop relationships among providers, and give patients a true voice in their healthcare system.

Healthcare, much like politics, is local. What we're doing in Yamhill County and in Oregon in general would require some adaptation if it were to be configured to the specific needs for other communities. At the same time, what we're doing here could work just about anywhere. A man slips on the stairs, falls, and breaks his wrist. Regardless of where in the United States this happens, the key issue is the same: Do you only treat the wrist, or do you look at the big picture? Our approach allows us to look at the big picture. It allows us to consider why the man broke his wrist in the first place, instead of just treating it. Maybe he lived in a dilapidated house with the electricity cut off and it was cold and dark. Maybe he had PTSD or depression. Taking care of him is a lot more than just setting the wrist. It's about recognizing and treating patients from a big-picture perspective. Since these problems exist everywhere, I believe this solution can exist everywhere.

Urban areas have unique challenges, given the larger number of people that are packed into a smaller geographic area. And yet, Oregon has urban CCOs that are doing similar work to what we've seen in Yamhill County. In larger cities like Chicago, one idea is that each ward could be its own CCO. It just depends on how one defined community and whether one can put the right people into leadership positions. Can it work anywhere? It can certainly improve things anywhere—that's for sure.

If you're concerned that the CCO concept might not work in your community because a meaningful percentage of your patients are of cultural or ethnic diversity, note that in Yamhill County, nearly 16 percent of our population is Hispanic. Hence, we consciously work to make our services bilingual and inclusive. Things don't have to be a one-size-fits-all variety. That's the good news.

So how does one begin? Go to the community providers— the doctors, the nurses, the social workers, the dentists, and so on. Tell them you want them to be involved in this process and take part in its leadership. They probably haven't had that choice or opportunity in the past . Trust the community to self-organize. All you must do is give them the basic structure, and then they can decide how exactly the whole thing will work. Reach out to hospitals, government officials, Head Start folks, and so on. The greater the outreach at the beginning of the process, the more likely you'll get buy-ins from the people you need on board.

Keep in mind that you cannot force doctors to do what's best for them any more easily than you can force patients to comply with prescriptions and recommendations. The process is not about telling people they must be a part of it; it is about asking people to join with others in the community. In Yamhill, providers saw the value of the process and platform, came together, and got the job done.

Another challenge in many communities is that the hospital systems are the biggest organizations in town. Sometimes, they are even bigger than local government, because they are often the largest employer in an area; they have the biggest budgets, the most revenue, the highest expenses, and the greatest number of suppliers. They may not be politically involved in a traditional sense, like serving on a county board or helping to set legislative policies. Yet, in a model like a CCO, hospitals run the risk of being the eight-hundred-pound gorilla in the room.

In Yamhill, we have been fortunate to have two hospital systems that essentially balance one another. One is a large, independent hospital that is owned by an out-of-state medical corporation. The smaller is part of a larger regional system.

If you are mulling the creation of a CCO, I cannot stress strongly enough how important it is for the hospitals and other frontline providers to be involved. These are the folks who actually see the problems, deal with the patients, and take home the headaches and the heartaches at the end of the day. These are the hospitals, the individual family-practice doctors, and other primary-care providers. In some cases, a provider might be the doctor, perhaps a nurse in his office, and his daughter working the front desk. In a CCO, the doctor's voice might carry more weight than, perhaps, the CEO of a multimillion-dollar hospital, because that doctor is out there seeing people and recognizing the issues. He's also the one who must meet the challenges of implementing decisions and find a way to get paid at the end of the day.

Don't be intimidated by the fact that large stakeholders may attempt to dissuade you from trying to start something like this. Do, however, involve them from the start, because their voices matter. Furthermore, and more importantly, in this model, patients—"members," as we call them—have input through a unique part of the governance structure called the Community Advisory Council.

If you want to create your own CCO, first see if there is some existing structure within which you could work. This may be a risk based contract arrangement between an insurance company and an existing Independent Practice Association of physicians or a county run clinic system. As I've described throughout the book, we had a legislative mandate from the state of Oregon to create this kind of change. Thus, we had rules and requirements about what was needed to create a CCO. In our case, the legislation specified a board of directors that would include at least one physician in active practice, at least one representative from local county government, and at least one behavioral health provider, among others. That set of rules gave us a basic framework with which to start.

Perhaps there is an existing set of rules in your community, or a stakeholder who wants to find a new way to deliver care. Perhaps it's an insurance company that wants to form an ACO or develop a new way to deliver care that is more coordinated in a community. If there's a simple framework out there already, consider using it.

If there is no such framework, that's fine too. You can still come together and use some of the elements that we have used, as they may be appropriate for your community. Just make sure that you are engaging a diverse group of stakeholders from across the community, including those who are actively involved in changing the "determinants of health."

These determinants of health include housing, employment, behavior, and education. These are the areas of life and the sectors of society in which we live and that affect our health during the 99 percent of time we spend outside a hospital or clinic office. In other words, you want not just medical-care and behavioral healthcare folks, but also individuals who represent the socioeconomic interests in your community, such as the head of a local Head Start program or people involved in transportation, housing, or job skills training. Perhaps you can involve someone from the local Department of Public Health.

The broader the representation of community stakeholders, the more likely it is that you are going to succeed.

I was a big proponent of including leaders from the various sectors of the community that addressed the so-called "social determinants of health." As a result, I was given the nickname "Dr. Determinants" for my willingness to embrace those providing "health care" but not in the traditional sense of being a physician or hospital.

In our model, the board of directors acts as the voice of the payer, because these people make decisions regarding rates and what kinds of programs get funded. You need to make sure you have a balanced board of stakeholders. The board needs to be informed by the care-providers . We do this by having a Clinical Advisory Panel (CAP) composed of different providers from around the community. They help set clinical policies and develop transformation programs to deliver healthcare in new and different ways. We also have our Community Advisory Council (CAC), where the members (the patients) or their family members can give input. It is really a three-legged stool: the providers (CAP), the payers (the board), and the patients (CAC). When all three are represented, the whole system balances.

To get there, you build an organization the way you would any other. We started first by developing relationships, understanding who the various stakeholders were, and inviting them to the table. Next, we generated excitement, showing stakeholders that a model of paying for and delivering care in a different and better way was possible. We then formulated our mission, vision, and guiding principles. This was largely accomplished by the CAC and the community members the organization serves. We then focused on metrics: How will we be measured for the sorts of care we want to provide? How will we meet those metrics and stay within our budget while living within the spirit of our mission, vision, and guiding principles?

Once we had worked out the basics for these issues, we had to provide to the state of Oregon, in clear detail, the exact nature of our plan for transforming healthcare. We addressed eight elements in our formally titled "Transformation Plan." Here are some of the key ones:

- Improving health information technology in our community
- Increasing the number of our members enrolled in patient-centered, primary-care homes or so-called "super clinics"
- Paying for *value* of healthcare delivery and not just *volume*
- How to address diversity: What were our plans for ensuring cultural competence, language training, and sensitivity to issues affecting different ethnicities?

It is an extremely valuable and necessary exercise to create a plan like this, because by doing so, you end up with a blueprint that everyone can accept.

We had to align our eight-point transformation plan with our metrics to make sure that our efforts would produce legitimate outcomes tracked by external parties and against which payments could be made.

Once you have these elements in place, you have the essential framework for a high-functioning, community-governed healthcare plan ready to bear risk for financial and clinical outcomes with a network of all kinds of providers ready to do the work.

It might seem absurd or unworkable at first, but this approach really puts the control of governing healthcare resources into the hands of people who live in the community and who appreciate those services—the individuals who are invested in seeing those outcomes. These are the folks getting paid for doing the work or receiving the care. To put it simply, this works and it makes a whole lot of sense.

This model presents an opportunity to move beyond what typically happens when an outside third-party payer—one that just wants to contract with doctors and pay for their services on a one-off basis—is simply repeating the same old song and dance. The providers are trying to negotiate for higher rates every year, and the payers are trying to increase rates on their members. The members, of course, are unsatisfied with the diminishing scope of the services they receive and the rising costs. In our model, we could provide an alternative to that unsatisfying and unrewarding situation. We now have a platform that works for Medicaid members. Yamhill could now potentially go and work with commercial payers and offer its whole network of services to commercially insured members so that they could take advantage of all the great services we offer, like our Persistent-Pain Program or teledermatology service.

Unfortunately, those with commercial insurance in Yamhill County do not have access to all these great services; at least, they don't right now. They do reap the benefits of these services because of a so-called "halo effect." That is, the different ways care is improved though increased screening, development of medical homes, and a focus on prevention apply to all members of a community. But the commercial payers may not necessarily pay for all the same services, such as access to telemedicine to which the CCO members have access.

A potential next step would be to go to commercial insurers and contract with them to bear the risk for the lives they must cover, so that we could offer them the services we have developed for Medicaid. Then we can also address the question that many providers face: What percentage of their panel of patients should be Medicaid patients?

Classically, Medicaid pays only about half of what commercial insurance pays, so many providers will limit their percentage of Medicaid patients to about 10 to 20 percent. As a provider myself, this is difficult to handle. One of the guiding principles of modern medicine is justice. Limiting care does not align with this principle, but, unfortunately, it is an economic reality.

With our model, if we can get support from commercial insurers, we can offer one single rate to the providers who contract with us and pay them the same for all the patients they see, including both Medicaid patients and commercially insured patients. We are then able to tell providers, we'll pay you the same amount for either Medicaid patients or commercially insured patients. We will measure your performance with both groups by the same set of metrics. You can then be paid based on meeting those metrics, so that you can develop programs, hire staff, and implement different resources to help you meet those performance criteria. These are resources that can then be applied across your whole patient population; you would not be offering these services only to Medicaid patients.

The result is a community where everyone has access to the same level of care—which is, quite frankly, how things should be. Again, as a provider, this is what I want for my patients and what my patients want for themselves.

Does this sound like a healthcare utopia? Not exactly. We still have our challenges, and we are still inventing and reinventing ourselves on the fly. The good news is that with each passing year, both our CCO here in Yamhill County and the CCO network across the state of Oregon are getting stronger, more efficient, and more effective. We are delivering better and better results to the people who need it most.

It is my fervent wish that you see something in our model that you can apply to your community. I would love to hear how things work out for you in that regard. And if you have any desire to come visit us in Oregon and see how we do things, our doors are always open.

There is not a soul alive in the United States who is unaware that we face a tremendous problem in terms of delivering and paying for healthcare. We spend the most of any industrial nation on our healthcare; one out of every five dollars of our GDP goes toward medical care. Yet when it comes to results or quality, we rank thirtieth in the world—and despite everything we've done, the situation only seems to get worse.

The approach I'm going to share with you comes from the state of Oregon, where we are perhaps more famous for fly-fishing or wine or our beautiful coastline than for innovations in healthcare! But I'm hoping that this book will change all that and bring to a national audience an approach that is proving itself in amazing ways in this beautiful state.

I'm a radiologist, which means that I'm a physician who interprets medical-imaging studies. I grew up in Valparaiso, Indiana, a small town close to Lake Michigan; I trained in

Chicago; and somehow ended up in a town in Oregon called McMinnville, in Yamhill County.

As a radiologist in a relatively small community, I started to see the same patients coming back repeatedly. I would see a chest x-ray of an individual who had congestive heart failure, and that person would be in the hospital twice a month with the same problem. I would sit there and do the best job I could of interpreting his exam. I would make all the correct findings and I would tell my colleagues—internal-medicine doctors— what was going on. They would admit the patient, and the patient would get some great treatment in the hospital, and he'd be discharged to his home. And then, he would wind up back in the hospital two weeks later.

I saw this not just with congestive heart failure, but also with so many other conditions. A lot medical folks call these patients "frequent flyers." It was just so frustrating to see these "frequent flyers" but be unable to do anything for them that could keep their problems from recurring, or could help resolve their chronic-pain issues.

When I started to investigate this conundrum, I learned that medical care affects only about 20 percent of our overall health. The other 80 percent is a function of things doctors and medical researchers call "the determinants of health." These include our behaviors, our socioeconomic status, our diet, even our education level. Since these factors that contribute to 80 percent of our health take place outside of the hospital, we doctors have no control over them.

At the same time, I knew there were people out there in the community—behavioral health workers, social workers, and others—who did work relating to these determinants of health. These individuals were trying to get people education, to get them jobs, to improve their mental health, and to teach them about their health conditions or their medical conditions so that they would not wind up back in the hospital.

As a radiologist, I had no contact with these providers. I would sit in a dark room and talk to myself all day long! It was just so frustrating. Many other providers in the community who actually saw patients face to face, such as family-medicine doctors, also had little contact with other medical providers and other community-based health providers. My wife is a local social worker who sees many of these same patients I do. Before the CCO, she rarely, if ever, worked with medical professionals on the issues of their shared patients. There was little to no communication among stakeholders and no shared mission and vision. Fortunately, my frustrations were soothed when I heard that the state of Oregon was adopting a new program to transform healthcare delivery.

When anyone in medicine or government hears about a new plan that's going to "transform" anything to do with medicine, the first thing we do is roll our eyes, and the second thing is inquire about how much it is going to cost and who is going to pay for it. However, it turned out that what was happening in Oregon *worked*. The building block of the program is what is called a Coordinated Care Organization, or CCO, and what you will discover in this book is how and why CCOs can deliver better and less-expensive medical care, to empower doctors, to get better results for patients, and to help "frequent flyers" get healthy, stay healthy, and out of the hospital.

To illustrate what I'm talking about, let me tell you about Catherine. Catherine lives with her family out in the country except for one week each month, which she spends in the hospital here in town. She typically presents with what is called an exacerbation of her chronic obstructive pulmonary disease and congestive heart failure. That's a long way of saying that she has bad lungs and a bad heart.

When she was feeling poorly and short of breath, she would call 911. An ambulance would pick her up and bring her to the hospital, where the doctors would check her fluids, give her oxygen, give her breathing treatments, and send her back home. But then, since Catherine was a "frequent flyer," she would be back in the hospital the following month.

Everything changed when our local CCO's Community Paramedicine Program got her an in-home visit to do a medication reconciliation and safety check after one of her hospital discharges. In other words, instead of Catherine coming to the hospital for treatment, we sent someone to Catherine to see what was happening in her home, and what our paramedic Tami saw changed everything.

Tami went out to the rural area where Catherine lives and performed a non-emergent visit. She wanted to get a sense of how the 80 percent of determinants of health were affecting Catherine's ability to live in a healthy manner. Right away, Tami saw several problems that were directly contributing to Catherine's repeated hospitalizations.

First, we saw that Catherine lived with her adult children and their families, and since there weren't enough bedrooms for everyone, she was relegated to sleeping in the living room on a mattress on the floor. If patients with congestive heart failure lie down flat like that instead of sleeping with their heads elevated, they are predisposed to going into exacerbation and developing fluid build-up in the lungs. Tami worked with the CCO to purchase an adjustable hospital bed so that Catherine could elevate her back, sleep better, and sit upright when she chose to do so.

Tami also noticed that Catherine's whole family smoked, and they would smoke in the house, when Catherine was sitting right there or sleeping in the living room. This was constantly exacerbating Catherine's chronic obstructive pulmonary disease. Tami worked with the family and counseled them, explaining that they had to smoke outside because the smoke was damaging Catherine's lungs, worsening her shortness of breath, and sending her to the hospital on a regular basis.

Tami considered the kitchen as well and discovered that Catherine's diet consisted mainly of canned foods, which typically have high sodium levels because sodium works as a preservative. Sodium is another trigger for congestive heart failure. So, Tami worked with the family to connect them to a local food bank where they could receive fresh fruit and produce, and not just canned foods.

Tami also noticed that Catherine's medications were a complete mess, scattered around the house in different bags and boxes. "Why?" Tami asked. Catherine explained that every time she was discharged from the hospital, she would receive a new bag of medications. She had some medications from her cardiologist, some from her primary-care doctor, and some from who-knows-where. No one was in charge. Catherine had no idea of what to take or when to take it. Our paramedic essentially organized those meds into a pillbox and instructed her on what to take and when.

All this sounds very simple, and it was. Catherine simply needed somebody to go out there and help organize her health. *The remarkable thing is that Catherine has not been in the hospital ever since.* She's living an incredibly improved life. She's no longer sitting in the hospital for seven-to-ten days a month and then getting sicker while she's at home.

The CCO is saving the $10,000 to $15,000 a month that Medicaid would have had to pay for her monthly hospitalizations. And our primary-care providers are no longer looking at Catherine with the frustration they had felt because, no matter what care they gave her, she just kept getting worse. We rectified this problem simply by being able to put boots on the ground and send Tami out to her home to see what was going on.

We're all humans, and all our bodies break down, either over time or because of a sudden event. When they do break down, of course, we want to be taken care of. But often, the reason for the breakdown is much more complex than one might imagine at first sight.

Take Dan, who lives in a boardinghouse here in Yamhill County. Dan came to the hospital with a broken wrist, and in the past, prior to the arrival of Oregon's CCOs, Dan would have had his wrist set and he would have been sent on his way. Instead, we had the luxury, in medical terms, of stepping back and asking the bigger question: "Why did Dan fall?"

It turned out that the boardinghouse in which Dan lived was dilapidated and old. The utilities had been cut off for a time, and the house was dark and cold. When ice formed on the steps, he slipped and fell. It's easy to say that the reason he slipped, fell, and broke his wrist was because of the ice—but the bigger problem behind the fall was that Dan's physical environment was very poor and a danger to him. This raised another question for us: Why, exactly, did Dan live in that sort of physical environment?

Because CCO networks include care coordinators, behavioral counselors, and other team members who are not medical doctors, we were able to get some answers. It turned out that Dan suffered from chronic depression because he had been abused as a child. He had never been able to complete school, get an education, and land a good job. So, fixing Dan's wrist didn't even scratch the surface of his real needs.

The emotional problems beneath his futile lifestyle couldn't possibly have been addressed by simply setting his wrist. Thankfully, Dan connected with a community health worker who supported him as he developed a personal budget so that he could eventually move into his own, safe apartment.

These real-life situations—the biographies of the patients, if you will—and not just the specific medical issues they were presenting, directly contribute to high medical costs and poor medical outcomes everywhere.

This is not just an Oregon problem; this is a problem that challenges every community in the United States, from small towns to big cities and everything in between.

The Coordinated Care Model that Oregon has pioneered—in which we bring together all the folks involved in different facets of health and all work under one budget—works. Moreover, what we are doing here could be done just about anywhere. That's what this book will show.

Keep in mind that we're not talking about commercially insured individuals, who typically receive insurance through their employer. Nor are we speaking about Medicare, which addresses the health needs of older Americans. Instead, Oregon's CCOs, like ours here in Yamhill County, primarily serve the economically fragile community, those who rely on Medicaid for their healthcare, to the extent that they receive any healthcare at all. These are the individuals who live in the shadows of society. They might not have any job at all. They live at, or often below, the poverty level. They live in situations unimaginable to many of their fellow Americans.

These patients often have substance-abuse problems and mental-health issues, which medical doctors, clinics, and small practices find extremely frustrating. They often "fail to comply" with whatever guidance their doctors offer, and from the doctors' perspective, they are often a drain on the finances of a practice. Medicaid reimbursements have been shrinking, and it's harder and harder for doctors to make ends meet while serving substantial numbers of low-income, Medicaid patients. Yet these are the members who need the most care, and providers need to devote the necessary time to address their needs.

Unfortunately, doctors, who have a personal and profession-wide mission to serve their patients, hardly have the opportunity to do so. They have so little time to spend with a given Medicaid patient that often, all they can do is prescribe a pill to take away the pain or lower cholesterol or blood pressure. They have the desire—but not the time—to get a bigger picture and understand why their patients are suffering. Without proper reimbursement, there's simply no way they can spend adequate time with Medicaid patients *and* keep their doors open.

The pills that medical doctors so often prescribe these days are opioids, which all too often trigger addiction. So, whatever problems the Medicaid patient might have presented—and as we've seen, those problems just barely scratch the surface of their entire health picture—now they can add an opioid addiction, which causes their lives and their health to spiral downward even further.

Catherine and Dan are not unique individuals. Millions of Americans live at the federal poverty limit, which is approximately $16,000 for individuals or $33,000 for a family of four. These are the individuals and families who qualify for Medicaid health-insurance benefits, and these are the individuals whose healthcare has become so incredibly expensive and unavailing to the system at large.

If you're a physician, therapist, dentist, taxpayer, policy wonk, or a legislator, and you're looking for new ideas about transforming healthcare—ideas that are proven—this book will offer you a new vision. I will explain why a collaborative approach works better than the traditional, disjointed system of care that exists in most of the United States. I will also show how the CCOs improve care, not just for Medicaid patients, but for Medicare and privately insured individuals as well. I will explain how the money flows from the federal government to states to communities, and how everyone wins, from taxpayers to doctors to patients to the government. I will introduce you to the thirty-three metrics that we use to keep Oregon's CCOs on track, and I will show you how we were able to overcome the resistance of the medical community—because the last thing most doctors want to see is yet another "sweeping solution."

When the Affordable Care Act was enacted, it essentially doubled our membership. I will explain how CCOs work together with the ACA. I will show the importance of addressing behavioral health and not just physical health, and I will take you through the Community Paramedicine Program that enabled Tami to go out and transform Catherine's life with just a single visit. We'll also see what the limits are to CCOs and how they can work in most places, with some variations on our basic Oregon theme. As you'll see, nearly 16 percent of our community is Hispanic, and we consciously made our services bilingual and inclusive.

Have we cracked the code on healthcare? Is this really the Rx for our ailing medical system? I'll tell you the stories. You'll be the judge.

CHAPTER 2:

WHAT'S A COORDINATED CARE ORGANIZATION?

A Coordinated Care Organization, or CCO, is a legal entity, unique to the state of Oregon, which gathers together various healthcare providers, including physicians, dentists, behavioral health providers, hospitals, and local government agencies, among others. CCOs bring all these folks together in one organization, with one common mission, vision, global budget, and set of performance metrics, to help them work together and jointly improve the health of a population within a community.

Stepping back for a moment, there are in the United States basically three different types of healthcare insurance. The first is commercial healthcare insurance, provided to individuals through their employers as an employee benefit or purchased individually through the Affordable Care Act's health-insurance exchanges. The second main type of insurance is Medicare, which is government-sponsored health insurance for the elderly. The third main type of health insurance is Medicaid—government-sponsored health insurance for economically disadvantaged individuals. CCOs deliver benefits for this third group, whose members rely on Medicaid.

I will discuss the flow of money in Chapter 5, but for now, it's worth stating that the federal government pays states money to administer Medicaid programs on a state level. Each state is responsible for administering Medicaid benefits to its own population. In Oregon, we realized that our Medicaid population faced some daunting challenges. First, the cost associated with this population was out of control. Second, the quality of outcomes was less than what we desired. Third, there was very little access to medical care for the Medicaid population because many members lived in rural areas, possessed limited transportation options, or had limited English-speaking skills among other reasons. Fourth, while there are many different entities paid to take care of this population, these entities weren't working together. We saw duplication of services, waste, and inconsistency. Yes, a lot of money was flowing from the federal government into our state, but we didn't see much coordinated management of that money.

Oregon's governor at the time, John Kitzhaber, happened to be an emergency-department physician by training. He, along with others in government and the medical community, recognized these problems. He also realized that the Affordable Care Act, or Obamacare, may soon greatly expand the number of individuals covered by Medicaid. With that, Oregon would be going from approximately six hundred thousand folks to over a million covered by Medicaid, which is, in fact, where we are today.

Oregon recognized that the status quo wasn't working. It was time to create something new. From the governor on down, we all needed to think not just about the individual doctor-patient relationships, but also the question of how the state manages the entire population it serves. How could we work with different local providers to get them to start thinking about managing populations, and not just the healthcare of individuals?

The CCOs that Oregon developed tied together not only those in the traditional healthcare system—such as physicians, hospitals, and pharmacists—but also community groups, public health organizations, social organizations, local government agencies, transportation systems, and even people from the housing sector. By bringing them all together under one organization with one global budget based in the community, we could coordinate care as never before—and coordinate payments as well.

Prior to the advent of the CCOs, the state of Oregon was paying a variety of different managed-care organizations, which served essentially as intermediaries between the state and the physicians. The problem was that all these different managed-care organizations were not working together. They did not have a common set of metrics. They would fight over money because they lacked a unified budget. By pulling everyone together, we could align our goals and work with each other instead of working against each other.

Another main goal of the CCOs was to develop a way to pay for healthcare services that typically cannot be translated to what is called a "CPT code". A healthcare provider will see a patient and then code that visit or categorize it in accordance with the CPT code system. That's how they get paid. Unfortunately, there are so many services that don't have CPT codes attached. We needed to find a more flexible way to pay for these other services so that we could improve healthcare outcomes and at the same time measure progress and maintain a uniform system for budgeting. What if we wanted to purchase a gym membership for an individual, or buy her a bicycle? How could we pay for problematic things like persistent pain treatment?

Many of our patients have persistent and chronic pain. Using the payment flexibility of the new system, we developed a multilevel approach that included counseling, education, and movement therapy. We buy yoga mats for patients, so that they can work at addressing their chronic pain. I can tell you, categorically, that there's no CPT code attached to the purchase of a yoga mat! CCOs give organizations the flexibility to dream up and then pay for all the healthcare items they see as necessary and whose medical value is supported by evidence.

Now, if you want to receive federal dollars for Medicaid— as do most of the states—and you have a novel approach that you want to try, you must apply for what's called a waiver from the appropriate agency within the federal government. Back in 2012, Oregon received a waiver from the feds to create its Coordinated Care Model and CCOs.

At the same time, we needed to act at the state legislative level to put some guidelines around these newly created legal entities. What kind of a governing structure should CCOs have? Whom would they serve? Two pieces of state legislation were then passed and signed into law by the governor. These allowed for the formulation of CCOs as legal entities and laid out specifics, including who should be on the governing board of a CCO and how to connect with behavioral health providers, dental-care organizations, hospitals, and so on. Obtaining the waiver from the federal government and getting the laws passed in our state legislature were the two big pieces of work that led to the formation of the CCOs in Oregon. Many healthcare leaders throughout the state played a role in this work.

Some readers may be familiar with the concept of ACOs or "accountable care organizations." These are, essentially, healthcare organizations consisting of hospitals and doctors. But we believe that if an entity is going to manage the health care of a population successfully and effectively, it needs to think outside the traditional healthcare system of hospital, physician, and pharmacist. It needs to work with a variety of different community partners, including, as I mentioned, public-health, dental care, and behavioral health agencies.

A CCO is a structure that allows collaboration among all these different entities and combines them into one system. You could think of it as a holistic healthcare system whose providers and leadership come from a broad range of disciplines that help to create healthcare outcomes—not just the traditional triad of doctors, hospitals, and insurance plans. This type of solution is also known as "collective impact," which occurs when organizations from different sectors agree to solve a specific social problem using a common agenda, aligning their efforts, and using common measures of success.

When your spending is governed by CPT codes, you are essentially paying for "sick care." We're able to focus in a much broader way on improving the health of our population and keeping its members from getting sick. One example is our Community Paramedicine Program. Another is a program to combat childhood obesity. A third is to turn all our primary-care clinics into what we now call Patient Centered Primary Care Homes (PCPCHs), which you can think of as doctors' offices on steroids.

Thanks to the funding we've received, we can hire folks called "behaviorists" to work in our primary care homes. We recognize that health is affected by our behavioral states; so, we've placed master's level psychologists into our primary care clinics. If you're suffering from depression or anxiety, or you have a substance-abuse issue, your physician needs to know about it. Typically, he doesn't have the time or, necessarily, the skills to help a patient with those behavioral health issues. He might have tried to refer the patient somewhere, but getting an appointment somewhere else is difficult. Frequently, someone drops the ball and the patient falls through the cracks.

By having a behaviorist inside the primary care clinic, a doctor who observes that a patient may be suffering with depression or anxiety can do what's called a "warm handoff," bringing the behaviorist to see him right there and then. Or, he can set up a consultation in that same office, so that the patient can receive behavioral health therapy in his primary care home. That's what I mean by a "team-based approach." Since we can spend dollars that, in the past, could only have gone toward physicians, hospitals, and pharmacies, we can act more flexibly. Hiring behaviorists to work with patients is just one such example.

When your thinking makes the transition from thinking about the healthcare of an individual to thinking about the healthcare of an entire population, you find that the questions are how you standardize, deliver, and track services. Many physicians tend to pooh-pooh standardization as "cookbook medicine." In actuality, there has been a tremendous amount of research and a huge number of validated guidelines for things like colorectal cancer screenings or screenings for abdominal aortic aneurysms. These practices are widely accepted, although some clinics follow them better than others. There's typically a lot of variability around how well guidelines are followed. If you're trying to manage a population, you must have good adherence to the guidelines, or it will be difficult to track outcomes.

Our Medicaid population has a large issue with substance abuse—both alcohol and drugs. Your doctor might casually ask you how many drinks you have each day. If you have some outward signs of alcoholism, such as jaundice or liver failure, perhaps your provider will ask you a few in-depth questions about your alcohol intake. Yet, as important an issue as this is for our patient population, a protocol for considering alcoholism or drug abuse simply wasn't built into the typical office visit. The 15 to 20 percent of our members who have some type of drug or alcohol problem were not well served under the prior system.

CCOs have metrics on which they are measured. These can include statistics about what percentage of the population is undergoing colorectal cancer screenings, or what percentage of the population has had effective contraception counseling. One of those metrics concerns screening for drug and alcohol abuse: the SBIRT measure, which stands for Screening and Brief Intervention for Referral to Treatment. It's simply a two-question document that has become a standard way to assess whether an individual has a problem with alcohol or drug abuse.

Previously, doctors may have only screened patients anecdotally. If they saw patients with signs of addiction, they might conduct drug and alcohol screenings. Since this service is now tracked as a metric for CCOs to receive incentive payments, we are able to get the provider networks to adopt a standardized method of screening. When patients go to any of our provider clinics, we hand them a sheet of paper as they sign in that includes questions concerning demographics, contact information, and all those matters. But now they are also handed another sheet of paper, the SBIRT, with its two brief questions to assess drug and alcohol abuse risk. Now, all patients in the community receive these screening questions when they show up for a clinic—not just Medicaid patients. Even folks with commercial health insurance or Medicare get this form. The platform of the CCO, developed to address the needs of Medicaid members, is now spreading to help the other members of the community.

Prior to the advent of the CCOs, if a patient did screen positive for alcohol or drug abuse, the provider often had very limited resources to help. Maybe he would supply the phone number of a local twelve-step program or he would prescribe some medication, but he couldn't really spend time to talk with such patients or figure out *why* they had a problem with alcohol. Do they have a history of abuse? Are they suffering from PTSD? Are they depressed? Unemployed? Does the patient have a developmental problem and can't read well enough to get a job?

Physicians often don't have the time or skills to determine the causes, but the behaviorists in our clinics do. They can discover those other behavioral determinants that might be influencing a patient's health and leading to drinking or a drug problem. We now have built-in therapy for several of these problems as well as a standardized approach to look for them. This model of care did not exist before the CCO.

CCOs can support high-performing clinics delivering holistic care because they are supported by the community and have funding to back the clinics. It's hard enough for a doctor to keep up with the latest developments in medicine. Asking her to keep track of developments in behavioral health, oral health, and so many other disciplines is completely unrealistic. To put it simply, there is a lot of stuff to know. A behaviorist or a psychologist is going to have a different set of skills and a different knowledge base than a physician, and will probably possess a different type of motivation to help people in those areas. Team-based care-delivery support, a fixed global budget, and the ability to fund these needed services with flexible spending—that's what CCOs offer.

When we first instituted the CCOs, we certainly encountered resistance from physicians, many of whom are very data-driven. They spend much of their time learning what lab tests can do and how to interpret the results; so, that's how they think. They think in terms of false negatives and true positives. As we shifted from stressing the health of an individual to stressing the health of an entire population, one of the first things we needed was data.

Getting reliable data regarding delivery of care to a population is challenging. Some of the data that we find helpful includes the types of billing codes that have been used, and how often each has been used. How many emergency-department visits has a person had? What are the codes for those visits? What are the dollar amounts attached to those visits?

In our community, we have fifteen different primary care clinics and about ten different electronic medical record systems—and none of those clinics or systems could communicate with each other. We had all this data, but we had no way to turn it into real knowledge for the entire community. We knew that, if doctors cannot get the data, they will be skeptical and things will slow to a standstill. So, navigating the data gap was one of the biggest challenges we faced early in the formation of the CCOs. As the requests for information came in, I became fond of saying, "Data is a four-letter word."

We were fortunate, however. We were able to get decent claims data, which allowed us to discover where we were spending money. We could tell what pharmaceuticals were being purchased. We could see who was going to the emergency department and how often. By sharing data openly and making it real-time and actionable, we could convince a lot of doctors that what we had to offer was positive.

Later in this book, we'll get further into the incentive system that rewards CCOs for creating better outcomes. The main point is that, in the traditional system, the more patients you see, the more money you earn. This is a volume-driven business and care model. CCOs, however, don't just pay physicians for seeing a bunch of patients for five minutes each. We pay them for doing things that produce beneficial results, like preventative screenings and addressing issues of behavioral health.

We also changed the way the individuals we serve think about health insurance. Typically, you might think about doctor's office visits, your annual checkup, some vaccinations, a trip to the emergency department, or surgery as the things that you purchase when you buy health insurance. Under the CCOs, we pay for all that, but we also pay for behavioral health services, social workers, and follow-up care after dental procedures, including dental sealants and fillings. When it comes to member benefits, we provide much more than traditional health insurance would—including the sorts of things that cannot be coded. For example, a child at risk for obesity can become part of our childhood obesity program called SNACKS.

Healthcare prior to the CCOs was "siloed"—meaning the different types of care were compartmentalized, isolated from one another. Healthcare providers who worked within blocks of each other simply had no way of knowing what folks in other community clinics were doing.

CCOs have allowed our entire healthcare-provider communities to come together, get to know each other, and unite under a common mission of working for and serving patients. In the five years since we began, the CCOs have become well-accepted. Forming organizations like this produces a lot of pride as different stakeholders come together. It's not just the healthcare providers themselves; we also have representatives from our county government, and we even have representatives from two of the major healthcare systems, which were traditionally competitors. In an organization like ours, we all can collaborate, and want to.

Before CCOs, many patients who lacked private health insurance were likely to go to an emergency department when they needed simple, non-emergency care—a huge waste of expensive resources. Part of the CCOs task is the process of education that extends to the patients, as well as the providers, about the services that are now available.

How do we measure the success of CCOs? There are two very simple parameters: one is money and the other is clinical outcomes. From a financial standpoint, we've seen our healthcare spending increase at a rate of less than 3.4 percent a year—a rate that is essential to the state of Oregon, because that's the arrangement we have with the federal government. On the clinical side, for the last three years, Yamhill's CCO has been able to meet more than 75 percent of the metrics goals set for us by the state of Oregon. We've received our full financial incentive payments as a result. I'll explain more about those later as well.

The CCOs have met both money and clinical outcomes criteria. From a financial standpoint, we are staying on budget. From a clinical standpoint, we are delivering an improved level of care, which is invaluable to our members.

The CCO consists of several different governing bodies. We have a governing board that broadly represents various community stakeholders, including providers of physical and mental health and representatives from public health agencies, local county government, and local hospitals. We also have a Clinical Advisory Panel or CAP, a governing body with actively practicing physicians, behavioral health providers, dentists, and social workers who talk collaboratively about various issues affecting our population. The third main body is the Community Advisory Council or CAC, a group where members or their families can sit, talk, and make decisions on various items that directly affect their care.

CCOs are not like traditional insurance companies. They do not manage Medicaid patients and dollars in traditional ways. The CCO is an entirely new method for organizing the provision of healthcare. CCOs allow for contact among a wide possible range of providers and other stakeholders, and allow the patients to be listened to as well. I call this approach "community-governed healthcare" because the community and the patients control it.

In the next chapter, I'll take you more deeply into the collaborative approach that CCOs create.

CHAPTER 3:

TOGETHER WE'RE BETTER:

A COLLABORATIVE APPROACH

CCO is essentially a new type of insurance program, governed by the community and created to address the needs of the Medicaid population. What allows a CCO to be successful is that medical care, dental care, mental healthcare, and even early childhood programs like Head Start all function together, instead of being siloed and isolated. Until now, there was never one single place for all these different care providers to come together and align their work, measure success, create better outcomes, and get paid to do all these things. The power of the CCO is its capacity as a structure in which all these providers work together, providing consistent care in a coordinated fashion.

When we began in 2012, we received some startup money from a partner organization with which to create an infrastructure. Think about all the departments of an insurance company. You've got a contracting department, a utilization review department, a credentialing department, a finance department; there are a lot of elements that most consumers never think about. But here we were, wanting to start a grassroots care organization that would basically act like an insurance company. We knew we needed that same kind of infrastructure.

For us, it was the classic business question: Build, borrow, or buy? We decided that rather than build all this out on our own, we would contract with an entity called Care Oregon, a Medicaid-managed care company. They did a lot of the administrative work for us. This choice allowed us to take advantage of their administrative resources and experience while we focused on strategy, solutions, relationships, and results.

Care Oregon had an existing presence in Yamhill County. Most importantly, they wanted to see us succeed as a community organization. They grasped the fact that, as a community organization, we were best equipped to make decisions for managing our Medicaid population. They also recognized that we would bear the financial risk for the care we helped provide.

Care Oregon recognized that, if we were going to start improving the healthcare delivery system in a challenged, rural area, we would need money to support those programs. They gave us a grant for about $400,000—money we called "transformation funds." That allowed us to create our "transformation programs" immediately and start impacting care immediately.

So here we were, a nonprofit healthcare organization for lower-income individuals and families, which essentially had to establish itself as an insurance company. We were now sitting on top of $400,000. One of the first collaborative decisions we made as a community had to be how to spend the money.

We immediately identified a lack of primary-care providers in the community as an important area of need—specifically, a lack of pediatricians. We simply had too many children for the number of pediatricians practicing in our county. When we first started, children represented about 70 percent of our population. We recognized that we needed to spend transformation funds to hire more pediatricians.

Our board approved spending a portion of the start-up transformation funds to help a clinic hire a pediatrician to see our members. This is a demonstration of the value of the CCO acting as a platform for broader transformation.

The pediatrician would certainly see the Medicaid patients, but the undocumented workers in our region also needed a pediatrician for their children. So, now the question became, if we were going to hire a pediatrician, what kind of clinic would hire him? This was a big decision, because it costs about $200,000 to hire a pediatrician, and that represented half of our grant money.

One particular clinic seemed like a natural fit for the new pediatrician. When you hire a pediatrician, you've also got to bring in a nurse, a medical assistant, additional technology, a reception area, and support for all those individuals and functions. This clinic had the physical space to take on more providers, and they had the administrative capacity to manage bringing on the required additional staff. The clinic agreed to take the money and hire the provider, which meant agreeing to support a team.

The challenge we faced was that, although this clinic was one of our larger community clinics, its physicians did not have admitting privileges at the local hospital and did not take "call" there. In the world of the physician, "call" is a contentious issue. Being on-call is a hindrance to leading a normal life, to put it mildly. You walk around with a pager. It can go off in the middle of the night and you're awakened from your sleep. Your whole family life is disrupted. You can't go out and have a few drinks and have fun, because you must be ready to take care of people at all times.

So, the first challenge we faced—the sticking point, in fact—was that we wanted the clinic to hire the pediatrician who would provide "pediatric call."

One of our two hospitals was located directly across the street from the clinic. When a child is born at a hospital, the on-call pediatrician needs to come in, do a physical exam to make sure the baby is healthy, and be sure there are no other needs to be addressed. That's known as "pediatric call," and it is one of the big responsibilities that pediatricians and family-practice physicians must manage.

Being on-call can have a considerable impact on a physician's life. The timing of childbirth isn't usually planned and often seems to come at a difficult time—for example, Friday at 6:30 p.m. The sticking point: Our new pediatrician would be working at a clinic that didn't take call.

We were the new kid in town, and we had to get along with everyone. How could we give money to a clinic for a pediatrician, when there was a hospital right across the street, if that pediatrician wouldn't take call? Our community needed an additional pediatrician who would agree both to see babies right after birth and to see children in the emergency room.

It took several discussions, but eventually the clinic agreed that the new pediatrician would take call. This might seem like an obvious step, but in the world of medicine—where things can be very political and personality-driven—trust when I tell you this was a very big step. Additionally, the on-call requirement made it harder to hire a pediatrician, because many physicians look for jobs that don't involve call. They want a normal schedule of working 8:00 a.m. to 5:00 p.m. in the clinic. Not all of them want to be required to come to the hospital in the middle of the night, especially on a regular basis, to deal with newborns or pediatric health emergencies.

In addition, if you're going to hire a physician who will take call, you have to pay that person more money. It's only fair; they're working harder. The good news is that we were able to resolve these issues in a collaborative fashion. Ultimately, the pediatrician was hired and we had a new provider in our community. As an organization, the CCO gained strength from its ability to support community dialogue on this issue. We became stronger for having gone through this challenge.

Having a clinic across from a hospital whose doctors never took call had been a sore point for years. The CCO was able to resolve a challenge in the community and, at the same time, bring in a new pediatrician to serve the community. To the best of my knowledge, this was the first time that leadership from different hospitals and clinics in our area came together and made a hiring decision for the betterment of the entire community.

Healthcare here is better now that we have an additional pediatrician who can serve our population. The hospitals are better served, because they now have a pediatrician they can call. The clinics around our community are better off, because they now have a place to refer their pediatric patients. The community as a whole is better served, because it now has more access to pediatric care.

Without the CCO platform and the dollars to support our decisions, the issue might never have been resolved or perhaps even acknowledged at the community level. We would still be suffering from a shortage of pediatricians, or we'd have a new pediatrician who would not take call, and the community's true needs would not have been served. People might have been talking about this clinic in negative ways, complaining that they weren't pulling their fair share. With the CCO, we could come together and address the problem head-on and solve it.

Another example illustrates how the CCO process was able to resolve a thorny issue in medicine while increasing service to the most disadvantaged members of the community. Most people are aware that there can be bit of a rift in medicine between traditional MDs and those who practice other forms of medicine, such as naturopaths, also known as "NDs."

Naturopaths are providers who have studied at a different kind of medical school, known as a naturopathic medical school. MDs study at what are called "allopathic" schools— and to complicate matters, there are DOs, or doctors of osteopathy, who study at osteopathic schools. In each state, each kind of doctor is regulated in a different way and is permitted to deliver different kinds of services. Often, the reasons for regulation are of political origin and unrelated to what will best serve the patients.

In Oregon, naturopaths have a considerable flexibility in providing care; they can prescribe many of the same medications that an MD or a DO can. They can perform a variety of procedures. In short, in many ways, a naturopath can act as an MD or a DO. This is because Oregon has a broadminded cultural outlook on medicine. We have a lot of people here who prefer to see naturopaths instead of traditional MDs.

When we started our Yamhill CCO, we realized that many of our members were enrolled for care at naturopathic clinics. This was largely by their choice. We also wanted every one of our members to be assigned to a primary-care clinic, and we wanted each member to receive an insurance card with the name of the clinic and the name of their physician printed on the back of that card. That way, they would know whom to call or where to go if they got sick, and they wouldn't have to go to the emergency room. They would also be able to receive the preventative care they needed, such as vaccinations, regular physical exams, and other services.

The wrinkle was that many members in our system were enrolled with naturopaths as their primary care providers. That may not sound like a big deal, except that Oregon's medical payment system classified naturopaths as specialty physicians, not primary-care physicians. Under the regulatory regime that existed when we started the CCO, we could not assign our members to naturopaths, and naturopaths could not be their primary-care provider. Instead, we had to assign our members to an MD or a DO and then direct them to see their naturopath as a specialist.

The problem was that we simply didn't have enough MDs and DOs to go around. We really needed to assign folks to the naturopaths to ensure that they got care, because for many of them, that was the only access that was available in the community. In addition, our members were asking for naturopathic care.

To address this problem, we convened our Clinical Advisory Panel, which was made up of many providers— physicians, DOs, naturopaths, behaviorists, dentists, and even social workers. We had an open community dialogue around the question of what it means to be a primary-care provider. In the end, we worked together to adopt a set of standards to define and credential primary-care providers. Our community's position was that, if a provider could meet these guidelines, then he or she should be able to qualify as a primary-care provider.

Our naturopaths now had an application process they could follow to become credentialed and certified as primary-care providers. All primary-care doctors—whether MDs, DOs, or naturopaths—had an equivalent path to take to obtain credentials as primary-care providers. Again, this might not seem like a major issue. In fact, it may seem like the most obvious thing in the world. But in medicine, nothing is obvious!

Instead of receiving a top-down decision by a board of tradition-minded MDs, the entire healthcare community in our county had come together. They recognized the value of patients' autonomy in choosing a naturopath as a primary-care provider; they did not want to limit our members' choices. They also recognized the fact that, if a naturopath can go through the same set of credentialing criteria and meet the same expectations as an MD or a DO, then he or she should be allowed to serve as a primary-care provider and to be reimbursed financially for his or her services at the same rate as any other primary-care provider.

Now we have some primary-care clinics that are staffed with MDs, others with DOs, and still others with naturopaths. It took a collective community voicing of needs and opinions to make that happen.

Prior to this new, inclusive approach, there might have been a Medicaid-managed care plan that would have decided to designate naturopaths as primary-care providers—or there might not have been. Again, it would have been a decision imposed from the outside. The beautiful thing about what happened here was that the community and its health providers could provide their input, and we collectively could make this extremely important change.

Elsewhere in the United States, there are insurance companies who are deciding to designate naturopaths as primary-care providers. These decisions, however, may happen in corporate boardrooms or are made by medical directors hired by the insurance companies. The communities who are served by these providers are not making these decisions. It's not the members or the other physicians, the peers with whom the naturopaths will have to work. These are privately or "publicly" owned insurance companies making decisions without community input. We'd like to think that our way is, perhaps, better because it allows for decisions to be made by those who benefit from the decisions.

Almost certainly, there will be those in the traditional medical community—allopathic doctors—who disparage the approach of naturopathic medicine. In our model, however, our naturopaths are expected to deliver quality of care at the same level as DOs and MDs, because our DOs and MDs have designated naturopaths as peers in terms of providing primary care. You can see how this changes not just the availability and delivery of medical care, but also the nature of community within the world of care providers.

Currently, approximately 55 percent of our members are children and adolescents, individuals eighteen years of age or younger. After the Affordable Care Act's expansion of Medicaid, the percentage of enrolled adults increased, resulting in a relatively decreased percentage of children. These children attend our local public schools. There has always been some collaboration between the healthcare system and the school system, especially regarding sports physicals. For example, if a child is getting ready to go back to school and wants to play football, he needs to be checked for a hernia and have a doctor listen to his heart and lungs. The school system relies on the healthcare provider community—the physicians—to perform these physicals.

In the past, there were many children whose families lacked health insurance or they had marginal health insurance and could not get their sports physicals under those plans. The provider community would, therefore, have different events where they would volunteer their time to perform free physicals. Now, with CCO and the expansion of the Affordable Care Act, most children do have sufficient insurance to get sports physicals. This minimizes the amount of volunteer time we need, which is a positive, because these are the sorts of things that insurance should cover.

We were able to take things a step further. We realized that, in Yamhill, because we had a relationship with the schools based on those sports physicals, we could use that relationship to address other kinds of issues. Our primary-care clinics, in conjunction with the schools and with the support of the CCO, sponsored what we called a "Teen Swag Night."

Our community clinics stayed open late one night in the late summer, before school started, to host the event. Typically, they close around 5:30, but on "Swag Night," they stayed open until 10:00. We sought to create a fun environment for teens, providing pizza and games. Various community groups donated "swag bags" containing T-shirts, puzzles, and other things teens enjoy. The idea was that teens would come in and get their sports physicals and then also undergo what we call the "adolescent well-child check."

One of the topics we'll discuss in greater detail later in this book are the thirty-three metrics we must meet each year for every one of our members. One of those requirements is that we do an adolescent well-child check or a physical on every one of our adolescents. It would be somewhat inefficient to perform a sports physical and an adolescent well-child check at two separate times, we thought—so why not just do both at the same time? Since you've got so many kids who need to come in for sports physicals, and they'll also need an adolescent well-child check, let's make it an event and get them both done at the same time. Let's also make it fun for the kids, so they'll want to come. After all, who wants to go to the doctor? But if we call it "Teen Swag Night," that might change everything.

It did. Our first Teen Swag Night was an incredibly successful event. More than three hundred kids came to five of our different clinics, both for adolescent well-child checks and sports physicals. We were also able to administer numerous immunizations. We found a lot of kids with gaps in their vaccination histories, and we got them vaccinated.

The event was successful because the schools got the word out to the students and were actually to create peer pressure . . . *to go to the doctor*. We were able to create a collaboration between the schools and the clinics to get these kids in and get them taken care of.

People often ask about the mechanics of getting events like these to happen. To put it simply, it takes a lot of meetings. We have monthly meetings of our Clinical Advisory Panel, the Community Advisory Council, the CCO board, and our Early-Learning Council. At these monthly meetings, sometimes our purpose is to inform, and at other times, it's to make decisions.

At a recent meeting, one of our topics was high-cost drugs. Several healthcare providers came together to learn about and discuss what we can do, as a community, to address this issue. Not only doctors were present at the meeting, but also behaviorists and representatives from early learning. Thus, all of these folks who touch on all the various aspects of people's health could strategize together to determine what we need to do in conjunction with Care Oregon. Prior to the existence of the CCO, these individuals would never have come together on a regular basis in one room, and would therefore never have had access to the same level of information or the ability to participate in community-wide decision-making.

We sponsor several community events throughout the year, and one of the biggest is what we call our "Pain Summit," for which we bring together all the doctors and care providers who help individuals with persistent and chronic pain. As I've mentioned, prescription opioid medications are a huge problem for us. The top ten drugs, by volume, that we prescribe in our network are opioids. Often, these opioids make their way into the community through diversion. The individuals to whom they're prescribed might sell them, become addicted to them, or overdose on them.

Additionally, opioids are not necessarily the best way to treat chronic pain. The individuals with chronic-pain issues who are prescribed opioids often end up with problems. So, opioids are a huge concern, not just in our community, of course, but also across the country. We wanted to address this problem by building some community awareness and talking about better ways to address chronic pain other than prescribing opioids. We brought in national speakers to talk about the problem as well as experts and leaders from the dental, behavioral health, and physical health communities.

One outcome of the summit was the formation of an Opioid Prescribers Group, which now meets monthly. They have adopted a set of common prescribing guidelines for opioids and have worked on developing a Persistent Pain Program so that patients with persistent or chronic pain can get treatments other than opioids. A community forum like our Pain Summit is another way we can bring all these different folks together to share information.

Another choice we made at the beginning, which I mentioned earlier and which has been critically important for us, has been the hiring of three bilingual, bicultural community health workers as part of our Community HUB program. They seek to develop relationships with our members and work to get our members tied into services. They are there to support members, as a kind of friend, and to help them navigate the healthcare system, a mission I can illuminate with a story

A few years ago, an eight-year-old child visited the emergency department three times over ten days to treat his "fever." Each time the boy's father took him in, the doctors who examined him recognized that the child did not have a fever. In fact,, they could find nothing wrong with him, raising the question: "Why is this parent bringing this child to the emergency department? This child is not sick. There's something going on here."

The emergency department referred the child to a community health-worker program, which is called the "Community HUB." The HUB has relationships with our primary care clinics, which also realized the child was going to the emergency department and not coming into the clinic. So now the HUB was getting messages from both the primary care clinic and the hospital emergency department saying that this child was ill. Was there anything the CCO could do to help? Should we send a social worker to the school? Was this a public health issue?

One of our HUB workers had seen the family a year earlier and could call the father. The father explained that his wife had been out of town, in Mexico, for two weeks and the father was at home holding down the fort by himself. He had never stayed at home taking care of his kids alone before and he was really overwhelmed!

It turned out that he did not have a thermometer in the house and he was very concerned that his eight-year-old son was getting sick. Since he was always busy working, and had never spent that much time caring for the kids, he simply had no idea how to detect illness in his children. He had kept his son home from school for ten days and had taken him to the emergency department three times. Why? Because he didn't have a thermometer.

Our community health worker gave him a thermometer, taught him what it means to have a temperature, and talked to him about other signs and symptoms of being sick. Then he connected him with a primary-care doctor so the father could take the child to that doctor on a non-emergent basis for a checkup. I don't need to tell you that this kind of care is radically cheaper, and a much better experience for all concerned, than going to the emergency department three times.

All this happened because of the collaborative communication between the HUB, the primary care clinic, and the emergency department. Because the HUB could reach out and work directly with the father—and buy him a thermometer—the system could save thousands and thousands of dollars.

It sounds ridiculously simple and, in fact, it really *is* that simple. When you start looking at many of these problems, you realize that so many of them could be solved with relationships and by just getting the right people talking to each other and asking the right questions. It's amazing how you can solve big healthcare issues—like over-utilization of the emergency department, at a cost of tens of thousands of dollars—simply by buying a two-dollar thermometer. Of course, not all cases are this straightforward. This was, by some measures, an extreme example of the types of issues our patients face and the solutions we've uncovered. However, in the face of many problem of the same general type, being able to uncover them and apply solutions has achieved enormous cost reductions for our CCO.

Prior to the CCO, there was no community HUB—no central platform, and no meaningful way to connect the primary care clinic, the emergency department, and the healthcare payer. The school would have been concerned that the child was absent. The primary care clinic would be asking why the family was not contacting them. The emergency department would be complaining that the child keeps showing up when nothing was wrong. *But nobody would have addressed the real problem.*

Now when there's a problem, a CCO member can go to the CCO, and the CCO, through its community health-worker program, can work to solve the issue.

When we rolled out our community health-worker program, we recognized that this was an entirely new way of doing business and a whole new model of care. Never before had physicians felt there was a trusted community organization to which they could refer patients, secure in the knowledge that that organization would truly follow up and find real solutions. There might have been a social work agency in town, and perhaps the physicians might have made referrals, but the physicians were not part of that organization. Now, the physicians are part of the CCO, are paid by the CCO, and help govern the CCO, so they have a much stronger incentive to work with us.

Of course, we had to overcome a great deal of initial skepticism. At first, there were not a lot of referrals to our community HUB. I remember thinking, why don't people just refer patients to this community health-worker program? This is a tremendous resource! We've got people who can go out there and work with these folks, take them to the doctor's office, help them pay their electric bills, help negotiate their rent, and provide all these wonderful services. But it was such a new way of doing business for pretty much everyone in the community that it wasn't used much at first.

I had to leverage my relationships with other physicians to get them to listen to the community health workers give brief presentations on their services. Or if I saw doctors in a doctors' lounge at the hospital, I'd ask, "Hey, do you guys refer anybody to the Community HUB?" I was doing everything I could to lobby people to take advantage of these great services we could now provide.

As a radiologist, I would often see imaging exams on my screen that I knew might not necessarily have been appropriate or needed. A classic example would be a young, pregnant teenage woman coming to the emergency department, and the diagnosis was *pregnancy*. I would ask myself, why is someone who knows she's pregnant coming to the emergency department to be told that she's pregnant? Shouldn't she be calling an obstetrician and setting up a routine appointment, and then getting a schedule for prenatal care?

What I came to learn was that young women in this position are scared; they're panicked. They'll come to the emergency department because they don't know their options. When they're in the emergency department, perhaps they'll get an ultrasound or a battery of other tests, and then maybe a follow-up appointment. But two days later, they're back in the emergency department, because they are still scared—and worst of all, they still haven't gotten to see an OB-GYN. Here we were, spending thousands of dollars delivering all this care that they didn't need.

If you're pregnant, you don't have to come to the emergency department to keep being told you're pregnant! If you don't have a support network and you're sixteen or seventeen years old, however, that might be exactly what you think you need, given the resources at hand. The individual can't be faulted for this. But as a community, we can recognize this as an opportunity to improve the options for these individuals.

With the CCO in place, things changed. Now, if I see an ultrasound pop up on a pregnant seventeen-year-old, I call the emergency department and say, "Why is she here? Why does she need this ultrasound?"

The response is often something like, "Oh, it's the classic story. She just found out she's pregnant. She's scared and she wanted something done, so we did an ultrasound."

"OK," I reply. "Did you refer her to the Community HUB program?"

"No, we didn't think about that."

"Well, that could be a good discharge plan. The community worker can call her and help her learn about signing up for Medicaid benefits through the CCO, if she doesn't already have them. That way, we won't have to see her back in the emergency department in two days and spend thousands more dollars to perform all this unnecessary care."

It really came down to reminding people of the existence of the HUB and emphasizing referrals to it. Over time, we've increasingly seen success stories like the ones I've described in this chapter. We now have more robust referral patterns in place. We're saving money where we should be saving it and spending it where we should be spending it. And that's a win–win situation for everyone.

The downside to all of this is that our organization bears all the financial risk for the care promises we make. Essentially, we're saying, "Yeah, we'll insure all these folks, and we're going to pick up the tab on all of them." So, we, as a community, now live with this financial risk, which is something new. When you have such a huge financial and social responsibility, it can create a lot of anxiety.

All the same, bearing this risk is a necessary element of the model. If we didn't bear the risk, we would not be as invested in making sure that the outcomes were good or that we were truly saving money. We probably would not be as motivated to come together at the monthly seven a.m. meetings to work on all these important issues. We know we're on the hook. We know that we must fund programs that will not only improve our patients' care and experience, but also contribute directly to our bottom line. So, we have to be very smart in the things we choose to fund and the individuals and groups with whom we partner. If the financial risk were elsewhere, we would not be as incented to do all the things we do to make this succeed. In short, we have a lot of skin in the game.

When new providers join our community, we must work with them very closely to make sure they're providing quality care that aligns with our guidelines and meets our financial-incentive metrics.

There are other issues that are less under our control, for instance, contract negotiations with the Oregon Health Authority, the state entity that sets our rates. What happens if government dollars dry up? Or what if there's a change in leadership in the White House or in Congress? What happens if Medicaid funding changes? Would we be able to sustain the current model under a different approach?

The answer is that we need to start thinking about how we can grow this model to care for other patient populations—not just Medicaid members, but also other members of the community. Can we work with commercial insurers to get paid for some of the work we do? Can we become a Medicare Advantage provider? These are some of the things we must consider if we are to mitigate the federal-funding risk associated with Medicaid and a possible change in government leadership.

So, there you have it. Whether you're an MD, a naturopath, a scared father taking care of children for the first time, a pregnant seventeen-year-old girl going to the emergency room because she doesn't realize other services are available, or anyone else on the healthcare spectrum—as either a provider or member—it's abundantly clear: together, we're better. The CCO is clearly providing better outcomes for our members and our providers.

In this chapter, I've given a few examples of this. The real question is, how can care get better for everyone? That's the subject we'll discuss next.

CHAPTER 4:

HOW CARE GETS BETTER FOR EVERYONE

We all like to talk about the U.S. healthcare system, but the reality is that the words "system" and "healthcare" don't belong in the same sentence. When you think of a system, you think of a structured, organized approach to performing a process for getting work done. Ideally, a system is designed from the ground up, with the end user in mind, and is geared toward a need to benefit that end user or to produce a product the end user really wants or needs.

By contrast, the healthcare system was never designed. It was never built with the end user, the patient, in mind. It just evolved over time. Some parts have evolved well and for the betterment of patients, but many elements of the system have developed for the benefit of physicians, insurance companies, hospitals, or other institutions.

The disparate healthcare system we have in the United States is not really a system at all. We have all kinds of providers out there—physicians, dentists, behaviorists, social workers, and so on—who have all developed independently of one another and, consequently, all have their own ways of doing things.

While there are some big hospital systems in the United States, there are still many physicians operating as cottage industries. One or two doctors might open a practice together. They might hire their spouses to work the front desk and their kids to work in the clinic. Alas, there's much more to creating a healthcare system than simply practicing medicine. There's population health. There's preventative medicine. There's screening for various treatable conditions and diseases. Nonetheless, not a lot of these things are taught in medical school.

When it really comes to providing for solid healthcare outcomes for an entire population, many physicians aren't equipped to deal with these issues. The way our system is organized—or should I say, *not* organized—our nation as a whole is not well-equipped to deal with those points, either.

Here in Yamhill County, we have about fifteen different primary-care practices. Before the CCO, as we've discussed, they did not have a unifying mission, vision, and set of standards for providing or delivering care. They all did the best they could. Perhaps the entity that most of these different clinics communicated with was the hospital, but that was only when their patients were sick enough to be admitted.

There were no rich conversations about how to transition these folks out of the hospital and back into the community or how to get them the follow-up care they needed. It wasn't really a conversation at all. It might have been a fax to a doctor stating, "Your patient was in the hospital and here are the medical records from that stay." Often, even *that* wouldn't happen. Prior to the CCO, it was common for a patient to go to the hospital and the primary-care doctor would never even know the patient had been there. There was little communication between healthcare providers.

When you think about a healthcare system, in an ideal sense, it ought to be *a system that keeps you healthy*. You would want a group of different providers all working together to ensure that you don't get sick, but if you do, they would all know about it, and they would all work together to manage you along the continuum from being sick to getting well.

If you're hospitalized, you're getting great treatment there—but what happens after you're discharged? In an ideal system, prior to your discharge, your primary-care provider or, perhaps, your behaviorist would be alerted to your needs and would become prepared to treat you after you've been discharged. As we all know, that's just not how things work.

The good news is that, with the CCO, we're starting to see more of a real healthcare *system* at work, where all these different providers are coming together to work toward the overall care of patients. One way we've done this is to create what we call a "Transition of Care Committee" within the CCO.

Transition of care is based on the idea that, over the course of your lifetime, you will transition from one care setting to another. Maybe it's from the hospital back out into the community, where you need to be seen by your primary-care clinic. Then the question becomes how to facilitate that transition of care from the hospital setting to the primary-care setting. Or maybe you've been seen in a primary care clinic, but you don't really have a physical health problem—in fact, you have a *behavioral* health problem. What does the transition look like between the primary care clinic and the behavioral health provider in your town?

As a result of the CCO, we can form a committee comprised of all these different providers, to talk together about what we can do to improve these transitions of care. An example of how a transition of care does *not* happen illustrates why this work is so important.

My father had open heart surgery. He also had Parkinson's disease, for which he had to take several medicines to control symptoms of shaking related to the disease. For the surgery, his medication was abruptly stopped in the hospital for reasons that weren't clear—probably because he had never been there, he had to have the emergency surgery, and the hospital never received his current medical records. He asked about the medications several times while in the hospital, but he was on several pain pills and, after asking a few times, he gave up asking. He just didn't have the energy.

When he finally left the hospital after getting great care, he knew he needed to restart his Parkinson's medications, but he usually had to ramp up taking these because they were strong. We were afraid that, after being off these drugs for several days, he might have an adverse outcome if he just started swallowing them down as usual. He knew he needed his neurologist's help in getting back to his previous level of medication. So, he called his neurologist to make an appointment. The next available appointment was six weeks later.

"Dad, did you tell them you were just discharged after heart surgery and you need help getting back on track?" I asked. Well no, he said—he thought they knew that. Didn't his heart surgeon tell them?

I had to hold back my tears. Feelings of shame, frustration, embarrassment, and confusion filled me. My dad knew how much I had studied and all the sacrifices I had made to become a physician. He knew how much I cared about quality of care and how dedicated to medicine I was. He knew my friends, who were also physicians, were the same. Given his impression of physicians and knowing how complex medical science and practice is, he figured that a simple phone call between the heart surgeon and the neurologist *must have* taken place. They were both his doctors, both taking care of him, right? He had just undergone a $100,000 surgery and had spent a week in the hospital. His specialists must *want* to make sure they are talking, so that he would have a smooth transition from the hospital, to home, to an outpatient setting. This just seemed like an obvious way of doing business, to my dad.

I asked my dad for the neurologist's phone number and said I would help get him an appointment sooner. He was still trying to recover. I couldn't bring myself to tell him, that's not how the system worked—that, in reality, there was no system. Yes, your doctors and their nurses and everyone else you've seen for care really wants to see you get better. They are committed to your health. But major gaps do exist that have never been addressed. No platform for coordinating care between these different entities has existed in communities.

This story was from 2011 and not in Oregon. Of course, some hospitals have social workers and discharge planners who help with these communications, but this is not the case everywhere. This happened, and similar gaps in transition of care still happen every day. Fortunately, with organizations such as CCOs, we have a platform to fill in these gaps.

To start addressing issues such as this in Yamhill, one big opportunity was simply developing relationships, so that each provider knew all the other providers in the community and what their roles were. In the past, providers had limited knowledge of what other players were involved in different aspects of a person's health, and they had certainly never met with those providers in person. It's not as though you open a medical practice in a community and there's a big orientation that introduces you to all the folks in your community who are delivering healthcare services—here are your behavioral health therapists, these are your dental-health folks, this is what your system looks like, and this is how information flows. Typically, nothing like that exists. But with the CCO Transition of Care Committee, we've been able to make that happen.

A significant part of our transitions of care work has been the adoption of an electronic health information exchange system, which we call an HIE, to allow information to be shared more easily among these different providers when patients go to the emergency department. Oregon and Washington together adopted a health information exchange system called EDIE, which stands for emergency department information exchange.

Now, whenever you show up to an emergency department in our state, that visit is recorded on this common platform, along with your diagnosis and any other related issues. (I can only speak to the process in Oregon, though.) A feature of this EDIE system also allows your primary care physician to be alerted to the fact that you were in the emergency department, as well as whether you were admitted to the hospital. Now you have a standard electronic information-exchange platform throughout the entire state capturing all this information.

The EDIE allows communication to facilitate transition of care. That transition may be taking place between the emergency department and the primary care physicians, or between the inpatient setting and the primary care physicians. CCOs have supported the adoption of the EDIE system and have paid for primary care physicians to be trained to use parts of it.

The EDIE system is designed to be used for everyone in Oregon, not just Medicaid members. Whether you're commercially insured or you receive Medicare, your visit to the emergency department is now recorded. So, the existence of the CCO benefits not just Medicaid patients, but Medicare and private insurance patients as well. By getting their primary clinics to adopt the use of this system, CCOs now ensure that primary care clinics know when their members have been seen in emergency departments or in an inpatient setting. You can see how this is a true game-change for both healthcare providers and patients.

Many CCO patients are economically disadvantaged, and some of them can lead transient lives. Now, if we have a member enrolled in our Yamhill CCO and she happens to go to Portland, where she is seen in an emergency department, we will know about it. We can find out what services in Portland exist to keep her from returning to the emergency department. It's also important for her primary care clinic in Yamhill to know that she's going out of the area to get care. What's going on? Has she left the area for good? Does she need to become a member of another CCO? Are our efforts with her still relevant?

Prior to the CCO, a person like this would be essentially lost in the wind, and continuity of care would cease. This was especially true for individuals with drug-seeking behavior, who might go to emergency departments all over the state. In the past, there was no way to monitor or measure such behavior. With the EDIE system, we could track these folks and could say, "You were just in an emergency department down the block a day ago." Prior to this system, hospitals and emergency departments had no opportunity to communicate this type of behavior—but now we can.

EDIE is a subscription-based service; you need to pay to access certain components of it. Some CCOs pay for primary care clinics to gain access to an outpatient component of this tool, which helps them manage their populations. Without CCO funding, it's less likely that primary care clinics would pay for that tool themselves. Importantly, by possessing the tool, clinics can perform better on certain metrics on which their pay is based, specifically those relating to the emergency department utilization of members. The information that we help them purchase allows them to meet their metrics, which increases this funding and bonuses. It becomes a virtuous cycle. We are helping these clinics to succeed by supporting their access to EDIE.

I keep coming back to this point because it's so important. We are seeking to shift the paradigm from simply the doctor–patient relationship—which, of course, remains incredibly important—to the overall community–population health relationship. CCOs pay clinics to manage populations, because if we're really going to improve healthcare and lower costs, we must be able to take advantage of tools that measure outcomes for entire communities.

I wouldn't say that these tools are accepted with open arms and that people cannot wait to sign up to use them. Sometimes change comes slowly. We must demonstrate to the clinics the value and benefit of these tools, so they can see how they will meet their metrics more easily if they have these tools in place.

For example, one of our metrics is the amount of emergency department utilization by members. Now, if you're getting regular care from a primary care provider, you're not likely to head to the emergency department every time you feel sick. You have an established relationship with your primary care provider. However, many of our members have never had a primary care doctor before. This is especially true for the more than four hundred thousand new members who have come to Medicaid in Oregon since the passing of the Affordable Care Act.

These newly insured members didn't know what it meant to be part of a primary care home. All they knew was, when they got sick, they went to the emergency department. That was the extent of their knowledge about healthcare. Many of them had never had healthcare insurance before. If we're going to stop people from going to the emergency department every time they get sick, we must help them learn what it means to be a patient.

We also have to identify when those folks do go to the emergency department, and have our primary care clinics reach out to them proactively and say, "Hey, why did you go to the hospital? Why did you go to the ER? Why didn't you just come in for a regularly scheduled appointment? Why don't we work on building a relationship together so that you can come here to get your care? We'll even provide you with preventative care so you can stay out of the emergency department altogether." Without a tool like EDIE, primary care clinics would never know who was going to the emergency department. Therefore, they could not initiate conversations like these.

Before the CCO system, Medicaid patients often did not have standardized screenings, causing a lot of issues to be missed. Another issue I keep returning to in this book—because it is so predominant in our state, and across the country as well—is the question of opioid abuse. In the past, we were trying to treat pain by prescribing opioids, because doctors didn't have time to treat the whole patient and see what was behind the pain or discover if there was addictive or drug-seeking behavior as well.

One component of the CCO-created Persistent-Pain Program is education. We teach our members about what persistent and chronic pain is, what triggers it, how to interpret it, and what truly works and doesn't work in terms of treating pain from a pharmacological or drug standpoint.

We also have a movement component to our Persistent Pain Program that includes elements of yoga, Tai Chi, and other forms of movement therapy to address each patient's specific complaints. Initially, this program was open only to our Medicaid members, but we've since opened it up to other members of the community. We are still looking for a long-term way to pay for it, but the thought is that we will be able to generate savings though less opioid prescribing and less need to manage the complications of opioid use. We see it as a valuable community resource that should be available to everyone.

Now, primary care doctors and even social workers are identifying members who have problems with persistent pain. By coming to our Persistent Pain Program, they can get treatment and avoid having to wrestle with opioids.

Another example of how CCOs benefit patients is, of all things, the use of flat-screen TVs in waiting rooms. I happen to be a patient at a primary care clinic in the Yamhill County network. One of the internal medicine doctors there is my physician. When I'm in the waiting room, I'll be sitting with other folks who have commercial health insurance, as well as some with Medicare and some with Medicaid.

In the waiting room are several large, flat-panel TVs. When I went in a few years ago, a lot of the messaging on the TVs was about the doctors who worked at the clinic. "This is Dr. Green. She went to such and such medical school. This is where she did her residency, and this is what she likes to do for fun." That's great; it's terrific to know who your providers are.

But when I went back there a few months ago for my annual physical, I sat in the waiting room and found that there were about ten different messages on the TVs promoting health screenings or other services that are in alignment with the CCO financial incentive metrics. Thus, you might be sitting there waiting for your appointment and see a message about the importance of having a colorectal cancer screening. The video tells you who should have the screening and how often, and suggests you make sure to ask your doctor—if they don't ask you—if you fall into one of those categories. Then there's another message about childhood vaccinations: who needs a vaccination and their purpose.

Now, everyone in the room—not just CCO members—are seeing those messages. These are important things for everyone to know. It's important for me to know about colorectal-cancer screenings, because the guidelines that apply to the CCO members are the same as the ones that apply to me. Prior to the CCO, that kind of common messaging wasn't out there in the waiting room. Now, we have one standard set of tests and treatments we're trying to get everyone to undergo or be knowledgeable about.

These aren't ridiculous tests either; these are basic practices that everyone should have, that are widely accepted by providers, and that are supported by research. Since, however, we didn't have a true health system—we had just a fragmented approach to doing things—we were never really on the same page. Now we are, and this waiting room exemplifies the unity of our messaging.

I also call attention to the link between our physical health services and our behavioral health services, which provide counseling for drug addictions and family counseling. Many of these benefits are administered by our local county health department, and another community partner provides some of these social services as well. Before the CCO, there was limited communication between primary care providers and behavioral health providers. These are two different fields with different communication pathways, different ways of doing business and, if you will, different languages. The common denominator, however, is that both systems were treating the same individual.

Since these two different elements of the healthcare system didn't know how to communicate or work well together, patients were getting shortchanged. There was often no good way to get someone from a medical practice to see a behavioral health therapist, or vice versa. Many behavioral health clinic patients had persistent, chronic physical or medical diseases. It was very difficult for them to communicate these issues to primary care doctors and get themselves into treatment. So, we developed a work group to address this problem.

The work group strengthened simple communication pathways that were in place before the CCO. There's nothing magical about the process, which utilizes simple tools like the telephone or e-mail—but being able to reach out to caregivers in a different universe of care, if you will, has made a tremendous difference in facilitating communication and in the handing off of patients efficiently from one type of service to another.

The Oregon Health Authority has supported the development of what's called "The Transformation Center." Its tagline is "Helping good ideas spread faster." It is a method of sharing best practices from one CCO to another around the state. Let's say that one CCO has figured out a great way to foster colorectal cancer screening for its members. This approach is taking hold throughout their entire community, and colorectal cancer screening rates are going up for everyone in the community, not just CCO members. The Transformation Center captures and shares information about this kind of success.

Sometimes there's a failure—a solution that didn't work. We need to know that as well. Innovator Agents are people who work with the Transformation Center to share information with CCOs regarding what's going on around the state. That way, if there's a good idea, we can all benefit from it.

The Transformation Center also established a fellowship called "The Council of Clinical Innovators." I was in the first fellowship class, along with twelve others representing CCOs from across Oregon. The idea was to learn project management, communication, and leadership skills, as well as to understand how to manage innovation and how to foster learning in an innovative environment.

In our case, in Yamhill County, we had only one dermatologist serving one hundred thousand people, of whom twenty-five thousand were Medicaid members. That meant there was practically no way for folks to get in to see a dermatologist, and access was even more limited for Medicaid members, since Medicaid paid less than a lot of commercial insurers. I learned this from our primary-care network.

I thought about it and realized that teledermatology could perhaps be a solution. As a radiologist, you could say I've been practicing telemedicine throughout my whole career. Essentially, I can log into any computer and access the PACS system, the software platform that displays x-rays from the hospital where I work. I can interpret those images from any computer, anywhere in the world, and enter a report. Whoever ordered the x-ray, or even the patient, can access the results through our hospital's electronic medical records system. So, I thought, I'm a physician with a set body of knowledge. I look at a picture and apply my knowledge and experience to interpret that image. I then make a diagnosis based on the picture.

It turns out that the practice of dermatology is very similar to radiology, except the dermatologists don't look at x-rays or CTs—they perform a visual inspection of the skin. They look at the skin and, applying their knowledge and experience, come up with a diagnosis and prescribe medication. Dermatologists don't actually have to look at someone's skin in person; they can look at a picture. In fact, that's one way dermatologists learn about their field: they look at thousands and thousands of pictures in books, in addition to seeing patients in clinics. Their skills in pattern recognition allow them to do what they do so well.

Teledermatology means taking a picture of a skin condition and sending it to a dermatologist so he can look at it and make a diagnosis. He can then e-mail the patient with a treatment plan in the form of a prescription. And with the issue of limited access to dermatology in Yamhill, I conducted a nationwide search for teledermatology companies that might want to partner with us. There weren't many, but I did identify one.

As part of my fellowship, I received a small grant in the amount of $15,000. I took that grant and purchased iPad minis and put them in our primary care clinics. Now, when a patient comes to a primary care clinic with a skin condition, the primary care clinics simply have someone on their staff take a picture of the condition and send it to the dermatologist over the teledermatology company's secure platform. Dermatologists look at the picture, make a diagnosis, and then send back the diagnosis and treatment recommendation to the primary care provider. It's really no different from what happens in radiology.

The result is that we've now created access to dermatology, not only for our Medicaid members, but for the other members of our community as well. Now, even if you're not a Yamhill CCO member and you go to our clinic, you could potentially have access to the system, depending on your insurance. You can see how this is a huge change and benefit, not just to our twenty-five thousand Medicaid patients, but also to the one hundred thousand people in our county overall.

The added benefit is that our local dermatologist is now more willing to see Medicaid patients and to see them sooner. That's because he knows that if a patient's condition has already been seen by another dermatologist—one of his peers—and they say it needs to be biopsied or needs a physical exam, he knows that the request is legitimate. He's more accepting of that referral and will be willing to bring those folks in sooner than before.

Again, we are creating wins for everyone: the Medicaid patient, who has better access to healthcare than ever before; the Medicare or private payer, who has access to services that otherwise might have been difficult to achieve without traveling a long way or spending a lot more; the taxpayer; and the healthcare system as a whole. The CCOs have ushered in an era that makes care better for everyone—and in many ways, we've only just begun.

CHAPTER 5:

FOLLOWING THE MONEY

FROM THE FEDS TO THE STATE TO THE COMMUNITIES

n 2011, the state of Oregon realized that healthcare costs for the Medicaid population were out of control and there was no money to pay them. At the same time, people on Medicaid for whom the state was responsible weren't getting the outcomes or the access to care they needed and deserved. That's when the decision was made to find a new approach to managing that population.

Oregon has always been a leader in trying to develop novel ways to administer its Medicaid benefits, especially in terms of managing and controlling costs. Two decades ago, Oregon became and remains the first and the only, state to have what's called a prioritized list of healthcare conditions for its Medicaid members. On that list, you'll find nearly every healthcare situation imaginable, from pregnancy to appendicitis, from sprain of the wrist to low back pain.

Oregon wanted to pay for care for as many people as possible, but in so doing, it had to limit the types of care it would provide so that those with more serious and more acute conditions—such as appendicitis or cancer—or those individuals needing access to birth control, would be served fully. The state wanted to avoid situations where people with serious conditions were not getting the treatment they needed. Prioritizing conditions would save money and allow coverage for more people.

Oregon was never averse to the idea of taking on big, ambitious policy and payment reform regarding its Medicaid population. The Oregon Health Authority looked at each medical condition and determined its severity, based on several parameters. If one condition scored higher than another, then it moved higher on the list. Every few years, the state legislature draws a line through the list. Everything above the line is paid for by Medicaid, and everything below the line is not. That's how the funding is established. The system allows the state to pay for more serious medical conditions and not pay for the less serious ones, which adds up to a better outcome for every healthcare dollar we spend.

In 2011, Oregon began the development of the CCOs or coordinated care organizations. In financial terms, the goal was to give control to local communities to spend as they saw fit, and to limit the amount of spending that was taking place—or, more accurately, to limit the cost increases endemic to healthcare. Since the money for Medicaid comes from the federal government, the state had to find a path that would channel those funds from the feds to the new CCOs. That's the process I'll describe here.

A federal agency called the Centers for Medicare and Medicaid Services, CMS, oversees Medicaid programs for all the states that administer Medicaid benefits. These states have considerable flexibility in terms of how they deliver Medicaid benefits and run their programs. That flexibility, however, comes with the responsibility to work with the CMS to ensure that strategies and programs will actually result in better healthcare outcomes without harming or disenfranchising some individuals or greatly cutting payments to providers.

CMS's role is to ensure that what the states want to do makes sense, to monitor their progress, and then to share best practices with other states. Oregon, therefore, had to sell CMS on the idea of the CCOs. CMS bought into the idea, but attached stipulations to enable monitoring of the clinical outcomes, because they wanted to make sure that care was really improving. CMS also set a financial target: healthcare costs would not increase more than 3.4 percent per year for the initial five-year period of the CCO model.

The good news is that we've been able to demonstrate to the CMS that our CCO model works. We've been able to stay within the 3.4 percent ceiling on cost increases, and we have been able to meet the metrics the CMS set for us. The amount of money that the federal government gave us to start the CCOs was a substantial $1.9 billion. That funding has supported the development of the administrative infrastructure of the program, to monitor and track it, and to put into place the necessary individuals and departments needed to ensure the success of the CCOs.

Along the way, we received a separate grant from CMS to develop the Transformation Center that I described earlier. The Transformation Center has hosted numerous learning collaboratives to help CCOs share their own best practices. It hosts a large, statewide annual forum and assists the CCOs in terms of helping them understand the various technical specifications of the different performance metrics they must meet to receive incentive payments. That annual forum has helped enormously.

Oregon reports directly to the CMS on a regular basis. We have to indicate how well we're doing on the performance metrics and also on the financial limitations we face. Twice yearly, the Oregon Health Authority releases a public report to the legislature and the media, showing how well we are living up to the various performance metrics from the quantitative standpoint. To illustrate the qualitative aspect of how we're doing, we share stories of improvement in care in those reports as well. Since we did not receive all $1.9 billion in the first year, we had to stay within those 3.4 percent guidelines to keep the money flowing. But we have, and it has.

When we began back in 2011 and 2012, we had approximately 600,000 people enrolled in Medicaid in the state of Oregon. Because of the Affordable Care Act expansion of Medicaid, we now have more than a million. We were concerned that with this expanded population coming aboard in 2013, we would see a dramatic spike in medical spending. The assumption was that many of these folks had never enjoyed the benefits of health insurance before and, therefore, there would be a lot of pent-up demand for care. Further, we knew that many of these individuals had chronic conditions that needed to be addressed.

We saw a bit of an increase in demand initially, in 2013, but by and large, we were able to stay within our budget and control costs. That's because the cost savings we achieved through the CCOs has limited the actual cost of care in the traditional fee-per-service sense. Although the population served by the CCOs practically doubled overnight, we could manage the additional members who came in through the Affordable Care Act.

The money flows from the federal government to the Oregon Health Authority and then to the CCOs. The Oregon Health Authority withholds a portion of those funds each year and uses that money to fund the financial incentive goals. If CCOs meet a 75 percent threshold of their seventeen financial incentive metrics, they collect those bonuses.

What kinds of metrics are we talking about? These include drug and alcohol screenings, colorectal cancer screenings, and diabetes screenings. The system was actually set up to create some competition among the CCOs, because the CCOs that perform the best on their metrics receive a larger percentage of the bonus pool. It's a new way to pay for healthcare. We're not pitting providers or healthcare systems against one another; instead, we're incentivizing community organizations to do well by the populations they serve. If you don't perform healthcare that's valuable for your members, you're at risk of not earning additional payments, which is known as an "upside risk."

In our first year, our CCO here in Yamhill County received around $1 million in financial incentives. Then, we had to make the most enjoyable decision of what to do with the money!

Should we reinvest it in the organization? What would be the most intelligent use of the funds? We convened the various healthcare providers within the CCO to determine what to do with the cash. The group decided that they wanted to see the dollars distributed to the providers who performed the work to help us meet the metrics.

Now, the CCO could have kept the dollars for itself, but since we are a committee-run organization that makes decisions based on input from providers, and even patients, the decision was made that the dollars should go back out to the community.

That decision could have proved somewhat contentious, because there were so many kinds of providers who could lay a claim to the funds, including primary care providers, hospitals, and surgeons. We realized, however, that primary care and certain medical specialties have been chronically underfunded in our community. Many physicians choose to go into specialty medicine such as radiology because it pays better and it's typically not as stressful to practice. I'm a radiologist, and this is what I hear from my primary care colleagues.

As a community, we realized that primary care is the foundation of any good medical system, and it is underfunded. Primary care physicians aren't being paid enough, and they face ever-increasing demands. We also realized that the reason we were successful in getting that financial incentive bonus was, in large part, because of the work performed by the primary care providers—not by all of them, but by a large majority .

Thus, we decided to take those incentive dollars and distribute them to the primary care clinics and our behavioral health providers, based on the number of members enrolled or assigned to them. Later, when our metrics tightened up, we developed the ability to reimburse clinics based on their performance and not just on the number of patients they served. Initially, however, we distributed the financial-incentive dollars based on the size of the patient populations. We knew that wasn't the best choice, but until we had better numbers to work with, that was the approach that made the most sense.

By 2014, we had received nearly $4 million in bonuses, and we had to face the challenge of how to return those dollars to the community. This time, while we distributed most of the dollars based on the number of members each clinic saw, we added the element of performance review. One-quarter of the funds was given to clinics based on their performance, and not just on the numbers of patients they served.

This was a challenging discussion at first, because some clinics were considerably further along than others in terms of healthcare transformations and outcomes. Some had already developed team-based approaches to some of the recurring problems that we saw regarding chronic disease, opioid abuse, and other important issues. They had more sophisticated data and better analytic processes. We decided, therefore, that we would pay everyone some money, but also reward those more high-performing clinics.

This is certainly a novel approach to distributing funds. If a commercial insurer has a surplus of cash, that money goes to the shareholders as dividends or to the executives in salary and bonuses—or the money goes to the hedge funds that own some of these companies. Those dollars won't go back to the providers or into the communities served by that health plan, and there is no input from the providers as to how to spend those dollars.

I'm not saying there is anything wrong with this. In fact, I will let you form your own opinion of the scenario. This whole approach—a community deciding how to spend bonus dollars to improve the quality of healthcare delivery—is quite novel.

I also want to clarify one thing about the 3.4 percent cap on increased spending each year: even though we are not dramatically increasing the amount of reimbursement, we are still able to deliver care in an efficient, coordinated fashion. Prior to the CCOs, every provider was, to a large extent, working in an environment lacking awareness of other resources in the community and not having relationships with individuals from other providers. That's a recipe for tremendous waste.

Let's take opioid abuse as an example. John comes to a primary care doctor before the advent of the CCOs and tells the physician he has low back pain. The primary care physician may have only ten minutes to see this person. John doesn't just have low back pain. He also has depression and high blood pressure. He recently experienced a death in the family and just lost his job. He may be very emotional. He may be unorganized in his thinking and unable to verbalize what's going on.

The doctor is trying to make sense of what he's seeing, when suddenly, the nurse knocks on the door. There are two more patients waiting to see the primary care doc. At the same time, he's being paged overhead because he needs to review some urgent test results. So, what does he do with John? He gives John a prescription for Vicodin to help him with his back pain.

The doctor has no idea what's causing the back pain and has no time to take a thorough history and physical exam. He has no other resources, like a behaviorist, to perhaps dive more deeply into John's problems and see if there are any other contributors to John's problem. So, here's a prescription for Vicodin, and off John goes.

Unfortunately, this primary care doc is the fourth doctor John has seen this month. It's not just about his back pain; it's the fact that John now has an addiction to pain medication. Yet none of the four doctors know that John has seen the other three and is getting all these prescription refills. No one knows that John is also visiting the emergency departments of local hospitals, getting more refills. No one knows that John is selling the extra drugs on the street, so you've got people out there overdosing, going to the hospital, and ringing up additional charges that the state has to cover.

That's an unflattering portrait of the system prior to the advent of the CCOs. The system is terribly inefficient, and one can game the system to further their drug habits. No one's really getting adequate care, and opioids are finding their way onto the street, where they trigger overdoses. Every year, nearly fifteen thousand Americans die from overdoses of prescription painkillers, per the CDC. John's scenario is, at least in part, where those prescriptions are originating.

It's not as though the CCOs have solved these problems, but at least we now have a better-coordinated system. John would be assigned one primary care provider. That provider would receive data from the CCO tracking the individual prescribing habits of each doctor. The CCO also provides information as to which of their members are on high doses of opioids.

So now, when John comes in, he's been flagged. He's been receiving tons of opioids, and there's probably something else going on—not just back pain. With the CCO in place, that primary-care doc can refer him to one of the community health workers, who can determine what's really going on. Is there a problem with opioid addiction? Is there some sort of behavioral health issue that's going on with which this person needs help? Does he need referral to our new Persistent Pain Program, so he can get education and training on how to deal with chronic pain?

The next thing you know, we've stopped the overprescribing of opioids. We're saving money on medications. John's not going to the emergency department with drug-seeking behavior, nor is he getting extra doses he can sell on the street, which prevents the overdoses we've been discussing.

This is just one example, but many programs are increasing coordination so that our CCOs can provide resources in the community to address a wide variety of problems. Put it all together, and it leads to cost savings and better health outcomes.

In short, everybody benefits—John, his community, and his healthcare providers, who could save money while providing more comprehensive care to him and others like him. The CCO also benefits, because by demonstrating positive results, it earns bonus money. The state of Oregon is pleased, because its residents are achieving better health outcomes. Ultimately, the federal government smiles on all of this, because it has the data to demonstrate that its money is being used wisely.

CHAPTER 6:

KEEPING ON TRACK— THE THIRTY-THREE METRICS

A lbert Einstein had a plaque on his wall that read, "Not everything that can be counted counts, and not everything that counts can be counted."

I love that, because it's a good reminder that, even if you're able to measure something, you want to stay focused on the data and the metrics that matter most. Healthcare is notorious for generating vast amounts of data points. The trick is knowing how to sort through all that and come up with pieces of information that show a difference or can make one.

The CCOs use a set of thirty-three metrics to measure the quality of care delivered, which, when combined with the costs, could show the value of care delivered. In this chapter, I'd like to highlight some of these metrics, because they illustrate the degree to which we've been able to increase the quality of care for Medicaid folks and, at the same time, have managed to lower costs in some areas.

I won't take you through all thirty-three; I could probably write a separate book just on that. Instead, I'd like to walk you through some of the metrics that tell the best stories in terms of the changes the CCOs have brought about.

The starting point is that you can't just demand performance metrics of people without asking why. There must be a reason for everything you measure. There's a huge need for medical care, and we're spending all these dollars. So how do we tell if we're getting value for what we're spending money on? Are we measuring the right stuff? Are we measuring things for measurement's own sake, just so we can say we are measuring things? Are we producing value with all these measurements, or just producing a lot of extra work?

Not only do we have to dedicate staff time to perform the measuring, but we also must create committees to review the data. Is it really worth it? Or should we just keep delivering medical care as we always have?

Four years along in our program, we've been able to demonstrate that the thirty-three metrics we've created are useful in terms of determining bang for the healthcare buck, if you will. Of the thirty-three, there are seventeen so-called "financial incentive metrics," where there is actual payment for performance—literally trying to buy better outcomes.

Often, accountants or other people on the financial side of things develop medical metrics. In this case, healthcare providers across the state of Oregon largely determined our financial incentive metrics. What makes these metrics so powerful is that they were developed with considerable input from actual, on-the-ground providers who decided what those metrics should be and how they should be recorded or reported.

Of course, there was a lot of skepticism when it came to trying to measure the results of our efforts. Once, when the CCO was starting up, I was promoting the idea of the CCO to a group of local physicians. I explained how we would better coordinate care, track outcomes, and pay on performance. It was very difficult for many of the physicians present to wrap their minds around what I was talking about. An older internist actually raised his hand and asked, "Is this legal? Has a lawyer reviewed the proposal for the CCOs?"

"The lawyers wrote the legislation," I replied, and I got a big chuckle.

But I added, "What I think you're getting at is that you feel as though this is being thrust upon you and you have no voice in the process. You're just being told that you're going to be measured on X, Y, and Z, and you might not think those factors are important. In fact, we haven't developed the metrics yet, because in this process, folks like you will get to contribute to the development of the metrics. Yes, it will take extra time and extra work, and it will take your commitment to this process. But this will really be your opportunity to have a voice in deciding what is measured and how the care of your patients is tracked. That way, when it comes to payment based on performance, you will have been an active participant in the creation of that process. That's the value of this CCO model. You, as a local provider—or even you, as a patient—will now have a platform to express what you think is important and to work on those areas with the rest of the community. It's not an out-of-state insurance company owned by an international hedge fund telling you what to measure. It's you being involved in this process."

I think he seemed satisfied with my response, or at least more open. It was certainly a big shift for doctors, most of whom don't like to be told what to do or how to do it.

So how do the metrics work? Each year, the Oregon Health Authority (OHA) releases a document listing the metrics, indicating dollar amounts paid out to each CCO for meeting those metrics. Let me give you an example.

When it comes to Medicaid, there's always a lot of talk about emergency department utilization—the idea that way too many people use the emergency department when they should be going to their primary care doctors. Unfortunately, as we've discussed, these individuals don't have relationships with primary care doctors and, so, they just go to the ED whenever they need care. They aren't getting preventative care.

One of the seventeen financial incentive metrics we track is emergency department utilization by CCOs. We incentivize CCOs by paying them extra money if fewer patients use their emergency departments. However, if you're going to get to the point where fewer people are showing up at the emergency department, you must build an entire support system to provide primary care and preventative care to patients. You must support preventative medicine and issues like colorectal-cancer screenings for adults or well-child checkups for kids. You must support screenings for drug and alcohol abuse.

When you combine these smaller components of the healthcare delivery system into one comprehensive approach, then you start to see a change in the amount of emergency department utilization across the state. Consequently, it's important to track emergency-department visits, because it gives you an overall view of how your entire health system is performing. If you have fewer people going to the emergency department, year after year, then it's safe to assume that more people have access to primary care, are getting preventative care, are not suffering acute issues to the same degree, know how to manage their chronic issues better, and get them taken care of on a nonemergency basis.

Emergency department utilization is a good snapshot of how the overall system is doing. From 2011 through mid-2015, emergency department visit rates for CCO members decreased by 23 percent across the state,[1] Obviously, that's good news.

Next. you have to tease out what the major factors are in causing that decrease. It's not always easy to tell. Is it because there are more patients in patient-centered primary care homes? Is it the additional drug and alcohol screenings? Are there more colorectal cancer screenings? It's probably all of that combined and the implementation across the state of the best practices of various CCOs.

Let me illustrate that point by looking at drug-and-alcohol screening in primary care clinics. Providers in the Yamhill CCO provider network now all have a standard process for performing drug-and-alcohol screenings on their patients over time as they come into the office. If someone is noted to be at risk, a brief intervention is offered in the clinic, often by a "behaviorist." Behaviorists are generally clinical psychologists who are supported to work in the clinic by the CCO. They have the knowledge, skills, and, most importantly, time to work with these folks to help them address their substance abuse issues. They also can help refer them to long-term treatment.

---

1   http://www.oregon.gov/oha/Metrics/Documents/2015%20Mid-Year%20
Report%20-%20Jan%202016.pdf

Another broad subject area we like to track is inpatient hospitalizations. When someone's hospitalized, of course, it's very expensive, and hospital costs are typically the largest part of any CCO's budget. Let's take diabetes, which can be related to obesity. Unfortunately, it's something that many of our Medicaid patients face. If diabetes is not appropriately managed, individuals are at risk for having acute exacerbation of the condition, which may result in hospitalization. They can go into what's called diabetic ketoacidosis, which basically means that their sugar and electrolytes are out of whack. They need to be hospitalized and have that corrected, and then they need to be medicated.

Hospitalization for diabetes is preventable if the condition is managed appropriately in the outpatient setting. Hospitalization is needed only if an individual can't appropriately control his diabetes, or if the care team responsible for helping that person manage his diabetes on an outpatient basis doesn't have the resources it needs. When control and resources are lacking, diabetic patients are admitted to the hospital, which results in higher costs for the CCO and poorer health outcomes for the patients.

From 2011 to mid-2015, across the entire state, we've been able to decrease hospital admissions for short-term complications related to diabetes by about 32 percent for Medicaid members. The CCO model not only reduces the number of people going to the emergency department, but it also addresses issues related to chronic diseases that can have acute exacerbations, which also would result in increased hospitalization admissions.

Thus, the question becomes, how do you measure reduction rates in diabetes? How do you create a financial incentive metric based on how well CCOs can manage diabetes? What we do is consider how well the CCOs manage what's called the "hemoglobin A1c," a measure of sugar in the individual's blood. You can track how well a person is managing his diabetes by examining the level of hemoglobin A1c in his blood. We track primary care clinics for measuring and checking regularly that hemoglobin A1c levels are appropriate, to see that diabetes is controlled, and we then also—and this is crucial—*pay them for actually doing this tracking.*

We are incentivizing clinics to manage the diabetes of their patients, so they're more in tune with the issues their patients face. Consequently, they can provide closer oversight and management assistance to these individuals, which ultimately results in decreased hospital admissions.

The clinics realize that we aren't asking them to do anything ridiculous. We're asking them to do something that they know they probably already should be and actually already are be doing. They'll respond, however, "Look, we don't just deal with diabetes in this clinic. We deal with kids who need vaccinations. We deal with people with high blood pressure. We promote colorectal cancer screening. Diabetes is just one of the multiple pieces of work we face. Can we get some help here?"

We now fund the hiring of additional staff in primary care clinics to build out a team-based approach to help with this. We're able to provide care coordinators and panel managers who can improve the quality of care for all patients—not just the diabetes sufferers. For example, panel managers can look through the list of all the patients that a physician will see on any given day and do what's called "chart scrubbing." They'll see that Mr. Jones is coming in, and he's a diabetic. They'll look at his last hemoglobin A1c, knowing that the CCO is paying the clinic to monitor hemoglobin A1c more closely.

So, let's see . . . has Mr. Jones had a hemoglobin A1c level drawn lately? OK, he hasn't. So, the panel manager goes ahead and gets that ordered and on the chart. That way, when the patient comes in, he'll go right to the lab and they can draw blood and figure out his hemoglobin A1c level.

Prior to the CCO, there was limited staff available to perform that function. Perhaps the physician would check, but it would be hard, since he lacked the support staff to do so. There was no metric tracking that performance and there was no money attached to pay specifically for positive outcomes. Now that we have this as a metric, we're able to provide better care for the many Medicaid patients who have diabetes.

This approach may sound great, but it still meets with resistance. I remember going to each clinic to discuss the metrics in 2015—we now have the resources for us to do this. At one of the first clinics, I met with their administrators and a few key clinicians, talking about the importance of the metrics and the dollars they could receive for meeting them. An older internal medicine doctor said, "You know, Jim, this is all great. It's wonderful. But I'm here to practice medicine. I'm not here to practice metrics. I want to practice good medicine. I don't just want to try to be meeting metrics."

It was a little bit of an affront, I must admit.

I responded, "That's all you need to do. You just need to practice good medicine. And if you are practicing good medicine, then it will be reflected in good performance on your metrics, because we're not asking anyone to do anything different from the traditional standard of care or best practice. We're just tracking it now."

Let's now turn to colorectal cancer screenings. Everyone agrees these screenings are valuable. The guidelines are very simple: If you're over fifty, you should have a colorectal cancer screening. In general, you can have what's called a fecal blood test done annually, or you can have a colonoscopy every ten years.

If you're a provider and you're telling me that you're practicing good medicine and providing the best care there is, then if I look at your patients, I should see that 100 percent of people over fifty have had the appropriate colorectal cancer screening. But if I look at the metrics and see that only 30 percent of the population has been screened, do I come back and say that you're not practicing good medicine? You're telling me that you want to practice good medicine, but I'm showing you data that suggests that maybe you're not practicing at the level you thought you were. This isn't an exercise to tell you to do better. This is a collaborative process to support the health of our community.

We are not trying to throw statistics like these in the face of good doctors. The CCOs simply want to help them elevate the level of care and the quality of care that they provide. That's why we come in with data and demonstrate performances of primary care clinics for issues like colorectal cancer screening.

We also provide them with the resources to help support those care coordinators, to help identify the patients who need screening. We're not asking doctors to perform metric medicine. Instead, we're asking them to perform the best medicine they can provide, which is exactly what the community wants to receive, and exactly what we want to pay for. By tracking it, we are helping clinicians do just that.

Our baseline data for the entire state of Oregon was set in 2011 when we started the CCOs, as we've discussed. In 2013, the Affordable Care Act nearly doubled the number of people covered in our state. These are folks, who, as we've seen, most certainly weren't enrolled as patients in a primary care home. If they had a problem, they went to the emergency department or an urgent care clinic. They didn't have a relationship with a stable primary care team. In 2014, our numbers that indicated performance based on various metrics in some areas in fact went down, simply because we had all these new folks and it takes time to get them all enrolled. By 2015, though, we were seeing increases in the performances again.

I'll illustrate how some of our metrics act synergistically. Developmental well-child checks are performed on young children to ensure they are meeting certain developmental milestones and to catch problems early. Doctors see children at regular intervals, particularly in the first three years of life, for developmental screenings to make sure they are progressing appropriately and don't have a developmental disability or disorder.

Prior to the CCOs, we lacked a single, standardized approach to developmental screening. Many clinics were doing it differently from one another, which made performance difficult to track. With the advent of the CCO, we adopted one standardized way to perform developmental screenings, in particular, the approach adopted by the state of Oregon. We were now asking all providers to use a standard approach to developmental screening at regular intervals.

As doctors see children more frequently during the first three years of life, they're able to determine which children have had their immunizations and which haven't. When children are brought in for developmental screenings, doctors also have an opportunity to address their immunization needs. By standardizing developmental screenings, we were also able to raise immunization rates. All the metrics build on each other. Now we're able to track it better and more transparently, and to share the data more efficiently.

It's one thing to get the data; it's another thing to have individuals who can interpret the data correctly. You also need to collect enough data in a substantive manner so that you can generate the reports needed.

When we were first starting the CCO, we frequently heard it said that clinicians make data-driven decisions. That is actually a little bit of a protective shield that physicians can put up if they don't truly believe in something. They start using language like, "Show me the data," or "Where did you get those numbers from? How was this information collected?" They start driving very pointed discussions around the data.

To me, this is quite funny, because medicine is two things: an art and a science. The art part has little to do with data. It's just based on individual experience, intuition, biases, and beliefs. So, I find it eyebrow-raising that when doctors disagree with something, they'll start relying on the whole concept of using data to drive decisions as a crutch, especially given that it is not entirely true. Medicine is an art just as much as it is a science, and the whole data argument can only go so far.

Nevertheless, many people were skeptical of the numbers we would provide. We would have dashboards showing how each clinic was doing, and even when the doctors had the data right in front of them, they would still argue with the numbers. That's why I often say that "data" is a four-letter word!

The good news is that we've moved along far enough in this evolutionary process of healthcare transformation so that the four-letter word around data has become the word "good."

That's because we're collecting data in meaningful ways and we're learning how to use it better.

Take depression screening. Many of our clinics perform depression screenings, but they don't code their work in such a way that it gets counted. They're doing all the right work, but they need to code for it—which requires a small change in an administrative process—to make sure that the work is counted. Then, the good medical care they're providing is in fact reflected in the data.

The challenge lies in teaching clinicians about this. Sometimes, physicians get a bad taste in their mouths when you talk about metrics or data, because they fear that it's going to take away their individuality and how they "practice medicine." Often, however, it requires just a simple fix on the administrative side, and it doesn't change the way clinicians perform their functions at all.

In all cases—regarding all thirty-three of the metrics—the crucial thing is that the people who have created these metrics are constantly reviewing them and modifying them, when appropriate. The healthcare providers of the state are helping in this process and have an active voice. Again, it's not some out-of-state health insurance company owned by an international hedge fund. These metrics were developed in our state, for our communities, and that's why we have achieved a high degree of buy-in.

It's even more gratifying that we're able to use the metrics to improve not just healthcare, but also other vital areas. While Oregon was starting the CCOs to address healthcare transformation, the state was also seeking to improve high school graduation rates, school enrollment, and children's readiness for school. The two areas of healthcare and education are closely linked. If kids aren't physically healthy, mentally fit, and don't have good oral healthcare, they're going to find the educational environment more challenging. They'll miss school days and they may not complete school. A lot of that is related to socioeconomic status, of course—the question becoming how we can tie healthcare improvement to helping young people get a better education.

After all, if kids don't complete school, and if they don't develop what you could call "health literacy," they won't understand their bodies or what wellness is, and ultimately, they won't have good health outcomes. These are the folks who will end up with uncontrolled diabetes and who will use the emergency department inappropriately. Thus, these two areas are very closely linked.

While the state of Oregon was fostering the creation of the CCOs, it was also calling for the development of another entity called "Early Learning Hubs," which you can think of as almost the education version of a CCO. These are places that identify underserved children in the community, evaluate the needs of those children and their families, and then work to ensure that programs and services reach and meet their needs.

The hubs leverage and coordinate with existing programs such as Head Start Preschool, relief nurseries, and home visits. They also work to reduce the duplication of services that can occur to provide the most relevant and effective services for families. So, their work in the education realm is like what CCOs are doing in the healthcare realm. This gets to the whole notion of working "upstream" to address health issues before they become expensive and unmanageable.

There is a story about a doctor who pulls two people out of the river and saves their lives. A moment later, he hears more shouting, and he turns around to see four more people in the water. He then pulls them to safety. Then he sees eight; then, sixteen, all going down the river. Finally, he runs upstream to see why all those people are in the water! Going upstream to identify and solve the problem is where we need to be. Sure, you need to help downstream, too—but working upstream will let you address the root of the issue.

It's the same thing here. We're trying to move upstream to improve healthcare, because a lot of the issues start very far upstream, indeed, even in early childhood. If we can get kids ready for school, if we can get them into school earlier, and if we can get them tied into healthcare services earlier, then we can prevent a lot of problems downstream. At least we can work to save them before they get out into the middle of the river and need to be rescued.

Here in Yamhill, our CCO is tied closely to the Early Learning system. Together, we identify underserved parents and help them get their kids ready for school by supporting them with different programs and services. We're also able to ensure that these kids are healthy when they enter school.

We have what we call a "Kindergarten Readiness Program" to support some of the mothers on Medicaid who did not grow up in loving and supportive environments and who, thus, never learned foundational parenting skills. Some are not sure how to play with their children in a way that teaches them to be inquisitive and interested. When their children begin school, they're not ready to enter an environment where they're supposed to be inquisitive, observant, and learning. It's not the parents' fault; they never learned those skills themselves.

Without any intervention, these young kids will go to school and they won't succeed. They'll drop out of school and have all the problems that come with failing to complete one's education. Therefore, we've taken on the role of educating parents on how to play with their children in a way that teaches them to be inquisitive and curious and how to pay attention.

In our Kindergarten Readiness Program, parents can come to a series of workshops over several months before the child even enters preschool. Now, these young parents can learn vital skills that foster curiosity in their children. Thus, when the children go to school, they're more likely to succeed.

By addressing the problem upstream, we ought to be able to limit the number of twenty- and thirty-year-olds who didn't complete grade school, who dropped out of high school, and who, perhaps, who have a drug addiction as well. We don't want to be the guy running out and pulling people in from the water. We want to move upstream, identify, and solve the problems *before* they happen.

As I said at the outset, I could fill an entire book on the thirty-three metrics, but I think I've given you a reasonably clear idea about how some of them work, and you can extrapolate from these examples. The takeaway is this: the metrics indicate we're getting better healthcare outcomes, covering more people, for less money—that's what this process is all about.

One of the themes I touched on a few times in this chapter was overcoming the resistance of some of the doctors with whom we work. The topic is so important that it deserves its own chapter, and that's what comes next.

CHAPTER 7:

OVERCOMING RESISTANCE

GETTING THE DOCTORS ON BOARD

et's go back in time to the years 2009 and 2010. President Obama had just begun his presidency and was setting his major policy agendas, of which healthcare reform was at the top of his list. There was much talk about the changes on a national level that would ensue. There also was a lot of misunderstanding among physicians, especially those who did not know what changes the Affordable Care Act was going to bring. Many doctors were skeptical that government would try to step in and control physician practices.

I would often hear from my fellow physicians that the government shouldn't be practicing medicine; that I know what's best for my patients; that those politicians didn't go to medical school; they don't know what I know; they don't put their names on the chart; they don't have the legal and financial risk that I have in practicing medicine . . . so who are they to step in and tell me what to do?

You could describe the climate in the medical community back then as at least highly skeptical. There was also a great deal of confusion in the provider community around healthcare. The Affordable Care Act was so big, and there was so much healthcare reform going on, that neither physicians nor patients really knew what to expect.

There were all these new acronyms as well: ACOs, ACA, PPACA, and terms like meaningful use, electronic medical records, and other sorts of things that indicated a sea change in the practice of medicine. On top of that, the Republicans and Democrats were spinning things in such a way that it was all but impossible to find the truth, or at least have a chance of creating one that made sense.

If you'll remember, Congress was hardly forthcoming with details in advance of the passage of the ACA. One of my colleagues compared the ACA to a kidney stone—because, to paraphrase former Speaker of the House Nancy Pelosi, "If you want to know what's in the bill, you have to pass it."

Here in Oregon, we were perhaps creating even more confusion by bringing the CCOs to life at the same time. The Affordable Care Act healthcare reform was happening on a federal level, and then you had the CCOs here in Oregon, which the ACA did not explicitly call for, but which were happening anyway. In Oregon, we had realized that our healthcare spending was growing and becoming unmanageable. We weren't getting the healthcare quality outcomes that we wanted for our Medicaid population. We also realized that, if the ACA passed, we would face a huge expansion of our Medicaid population—which is exactly what happened. So, we had to act.

In Yamhill County, there was a lot of confusion among physicians about the various terms and concepts. What's the Affordable Care Act? What's Obamacare? What are Coordinated Care Organizations? Many physicians actually lacked the basic understanding of the difference between Medicaid and Medicare, especially the creatively named and completely non-descriptive four components of Medicare: Parts A, B, C, & D.

Let's take a step back. For physicians, four basic ethical principles guide modern American medicine. The first is *autonomy*, which means that patients should have a right to make their own decisions regarding treatment. They shouldn't be coerced into a treatment or told what they need to have done. They should be given the facts, along with some guidance from their physician, but it shouldn't be the physician telling them what must happen next.

The second concept is *beneficence*, meaning that the treatments you deliver are intended to produce good outcomes or, at least, a better result than what the patient is currently experiencing.

The third is *nonmaleficence*, which basically refers to the "first, do no harm" concept enshrined in the Hippocratic Oath: Don't do anything that's going to hurt a person.

The fourth major tenet is *justice*, which means, basically, that medical care should be fair. There are different interpretations of this concept, but it essentially refers to the idea that all individuals should have just and equal access to medical treatment, regardless of who the payer is and without consideration of their socioeconomic status, race, ethnicity, gender, age, and more. You might be a billionaire who's independently insured, or you might be a Medicaid member. But if you have a cough and a fever and it's three in the morning, and you go to the emergency department, you should have equal access to a chest x-ray—no matter who will be paying. It doesn't mean that the billionaire gets the chest x-ray and the poor Medicaid member does not.

At the same time, in addition to these four tenets, physicians also run businesses. They have to earn money, keep the lights on, and pay staff. That means many decisions must be made in the business realm and not just the realm of care, which brings us to Medicare and Medicaid.

Remember that doctors are already tasked with knowing so much medical information and must deal with the emotional burden and the psychological issues that their patients bring to the table. On top of that, there is a whole additional layer of bureaucracy, government regulations, and business models. It is almost too much for most people, even doctors, to handle.

In the year or so prior to the passage of the ACA, there was so much going on that physicians were just throwing up their hands and saying, "I'm just going to practice medicine the way I've always done it. The government is not going to tell me what to do. I'm not going to follow any metrics. The people are going to pay me what I demand. If I don't want to take any patients, I don't have to. I'm my own boss."

This gets to the fact that much of medicine is still a cottage industry, almost a mom-and-pop–type industry, although that is changing. Hospitals or large medical practices now employ more than 60 percent of all physicians,[2] which is the greatest percentage in U.S. history. Yet, there is a saying: "You can employ physicians, but that doesn't make them employees." Even though you're paying them, it doesn't necessarily mean that they're going to do everything you say.

Against this complex and confusing backdrop, the CCOs came into existence. I didn't see the CCOs as a big-government initiative trying to come in and tell doctors what to do, or telling them that they had to see Medicaid patients and this is what they were going to get paid, or that they would have to meet these metrics. Instead, I saw the CCOs as an opportunity to create a community organization to govern the healthcare resources available in our community.

It wasn't big government stepping in to command, "You have to do this." Instead, it was big government saying, "Hey, local community, local physicians, here's your platform. Here's your opportunity to control your own destiny. If you guys build a CCO, if you're willing to bear the financial risk and the quality risk for the care you deliver, then go for it. We'll pay you a global budget. We'll give you the money. Then, you guys can set your rates, and you can decide how you're going to manage the quality in the outcomes. Yes, we'll set the metrics, and we've got specific benchmarks that we want you to meet, but it's up to you to figure out how you're going to get there." That was a lot more palatable to me, and when I had a chance to explain it to doctors in these terms, it was a lot more acceptable to them as well.

Since doctors don't like to be told what to do, you can certainly imagine that, when we introduced all these metrics,

---

2   Katie Sullivan. "Is physician employment the right move for hospitals?" http://www.fiercehealthcare.com /story/physician-employment-right-move-hospitals/2014-05-28

they were less than enthused. That's especially the case because this was happening against the backdrop of the ACA, which threatened to change everything.

One of the financial incentive metrics put forth by the state of Oregon was that all CCOs had to perform adolescent well-child checks on a certain number of individuals. At first, providers were resistant, saying, "This is silly. Why is the government telling me I have to do this?"

So, we responded, "If we look at the adolescent population in Oregon, we have the second lowest high school graduation rate in the United States.[3] We're also in the top ten in terms of adolescent suicides, and in the top six in terms of adolescent drug abuse.[4] Our adolescent population in Oregon faces exceptional challenges. Thus, it makes total sense that we, as healthcare providers—we, as individuals responsible for these people's health—should be seeing adolescents once a year. They're vulnerable. We should check in on what they're doing."

When we put it that way, it made sense. The things the state of Oregon was asking doctors to do were not unrealistic. In fact, they were extremely rational. The state was saying, "Build your CCO and then figure out how you want to conduct adolescent well-child checks." That's when we created that event we called the Teen Swag Night, as I explained. We had the freedom to create the program as we saw fit, and not just on terms dictated by the government.

As long as the ask was clear—as in, "Hey, providers, you need to do X number of adolescent well-child checks a year"—that cut through a lot of the confusion, and confusion was the source of much of the resistance. When you ask doctors to do

---

3   http://www.governing.com/gov-data/high-school-graduation-rates-by-state.html
4   http://archive.samhsa.gov/data/NSDUH/2k11State/NSDUHsaeTables2011.pdf

something that makes total sense, they typically say, "Hey, this should've been happening all along."

We are now doing more adolescent well-child checks than ever. The state gave providers a new level of autonomy, a framework to function within, and the ability to control their own destiny. Obamacare didn't come in and say, "Once a year, on a Wednesday night, you have to have a Teen Swag Night, give out pizza, and perform vaccinations." That would be ridiculous. There's nothing like that in the Affordable Care Act.

Rather, here in Oregon, with our Coordinated Care Model, we've created a structure that allows communities to decide how they want to go about getting kids in for immunizations. That sort of professional energy might not have been expended in these positive ways prior to the CCOs. You can say we got ourselves "Oregon-ized."

Aside from the metrics, the financial risk was also an obstacle when we were trying to get doctors to buy into the CCOs. Typically, we would talk to physicians about financial risk and they would say, "Oh, capitated care—back in the 1990s, we all lost our shirts on this. This isn't going to work."

However, that was a different model back then; now the financial risk borne by providers takes place at the level of the organization—at the level of the CCO community. So, the doctors themselves don't bear financial risk. If anyone gets into trouble, it would be the CCO, not the doctor.

We do have financial reserves to safeguard against as well as reinsurance. If we have a few high-cost cases in the millions of dollars that could potentially bust our budget, we have limited our risk. Reinsurance will kick in and pay for those extremely rare, high-cost cases, if they come along. Learning how to better safeguard against that risk was something new and different that the CCOs offered.

We've talked elsewhere in this book about Accountable Care Organizations or ACOs, which are healthcare system–focused; these were initiatives developed through the Affordable Care Act. We had attempted to start an ACO in Yamhill County. It was unsuccessful for a variety of reasons. Reflecting on it now, it's easy to see why the CCO model has been successful and the ACO completely failed here.

The CCO brings in stakeholders from across the community; it's not just the hospital and the physicians at the table. With the CCO, as we've discussed, it's also the local county government, the local department of public health, the local community-service organizations, our local community behavioral health providers, our local dental organizations, and our early-learning system with our Head Start program. It was really a much bigger, richer organization than the ACO, which was focused strictly on the hospitals and doctors and was, to some extent, motivated by profit.

As we've reviewed earlier, for the average individual, only 20 percent of health is a function of medical care; other factors determine the other 80 percent, factors including housing, education, economic status, and behaviors. You're naturally going to be much more successful if you are organizing an entity that affects all the factors that determine health, and not just medical care. That's why the CCOs have worked.

At the time, the attempted local ACO was billed as an opportunity for doctors to make a lot of money—but it failed, perhaps because it was overly focused on making money. The ACOs were largely about creating a market share, as far as I could tell, and trying to bring in a lot of commercially insured patients. They were not focused on the whole community or on bringing all the constituent elements together to create a better working environment. Ultimately, that's why the CCO model has worked so much better.

It sounds so Pollyanna-ish or "pie in the sky" to say that, if you bring folks together to address and assist the most vulnerable members of society, you'll develop better healthcare. Of course, people would be skeptical, but the proof of the pudding is in the eating, and the metrics don't lie. We really are providing better healthcare to more people who would not have gotten access to care in the past.

It's very satisfying for all of us to know that we're making a difference in the lives of so many people. On a personal level, knowing I've helped establish the CCOs means more to me than the idea of getting paid a lot more money for reading more MRIs.

Obviously, money is a very important matter for doctors. Healthcare payments are in a state of disorder. Some providers have capitated contracts, which are essentially risk arrangements where they bear the full financial risk. By and large, however, in the United States, medical care exists in a fee-for-service environment.

A doctor sees a patient and then submits a bill based on what's called a "CPT code" that is assigned a relative value unit, or RVU. I could get into the details of RVUs and conversion factors, but doctors reading this book already know what I'm talking about. The result is that most doctors are paid for the volume of services they perform.

Physicians were comfortable with this system, as they knew that the harder they worked, and the more work they did, the more they would get paid. The problem is that a system that rewards seeing high numbers of patients practically guarantees that few, if any, of those patients will get great care. Physicians would see a lot of people, but did they really make the right diagnoses? Did they really give them the right treatment?

Often, if you didn't make the right diagnosis or provide the right treatment, you would be paid more, because those people would come back and you'd need to see them again. The system doesn't really pay for quality; that's a downside of the fee-for-service approach. On the flip side, with capitation, if someone is really sick but the physician is only receiving a capitated rate of $100 a month, he is going to lose a ton of money by spending so much time with one person.

Thus, while doctors were certainly skeptical about the CCOs and the potential changes in the payment system, deep down, they knew that it wasn't the best system because it didn't necessarily promote the best outcomes. We are by no means finished getting the payment model perfect, but we've been able to create what we call a value-based payment model for our primary care clinics, one that is better than anything that has come along so far.

Let me explain how it works.

The value-based payment model combines fee-for-service along with a performance-based payment. The approach was developed in partnership with our providers and administrators for major clinics. If you think about it, it's pretty amazing that they would all sit down to work with a payer. What health plan actually allows the providers to come up with the payment mechanism?

Typically, a commercial insurer sends you, as a provider, a contract and says, "Here's your conversion rate. We'll pay you $100 at this conversion rate, then you multiply your RVUs by that conversion rate, and that's what you'll get paid." There's no negotiation, and, typically, it's an "evergreen" contract, which means it rolls over each year with no input from the providers. Payers in this model are not necessarily interested in quality; they just want to keep costs down.

In our model, we work with the providers to develop a payment system that makes sense for them but also pays based on quality and performance, making sense thereby for our members as well. We're paying fee-for-service rates, but we add to this a value-based component. To put it simply, if your clinic meets certain quality metrics, you'll receive an additional dollar amount for each member you have enrolled. For example, if you meet a determined benchmark from the state of Oregon for the number of colorectal cancer screenings your patients have had, you'll make more money.

Here's an example: If you have one thousand members and the benchmark for colorectal-cancer screenings is 80 percent of those members, and if you do colorectal-cancer screenings on 85 percent of them, you'll get $1 per member per month or an additional $1,000 per month for meeting that benchmark. When asked us to come up with a way to incentivize clinics to meet their metrics, we came up with this per-member-per-month add-on rate. It encourages clinics to get to that benchmark and stay there, because if they fall short of the benchmark, they'll lose on those additional payments and they don't want that to happen.

To make sure that the clinics understood the necessary work to receive those additional amounts, we set up a facilitated primary care collaborative group. Each month, all our primary care clinics would come together in an organized, structured fashion to talk about metrics. Each month, the group would focus on one or two metrics and discuss best practices, what works, and so on. This keeps the excitement and interest going, and it also allows clinics to learn about local resources and build relationships. We can find out what's worked for one clinic in terms of, say, getting information out of their electronic medical-records system, or working with the CCOs to get that information. Now, this is tough because it takes time out of the day. You've got to commit staff to go to these meetings to learn about these things. But the payments are there, so if you're willing to put in the work, and willing to commit to delivering higher-quality care, then you can benefit financially.

Most of our initial efforts regarding the value-based payment model have focused on primary care. The next step will be working with specialists, which is going to be more challenging. We'll most likely begin by determining the most expensive specialties and discovering which ones are costliest for the CCOs.

Most likely, the list will include my specialty, radiology, because one of the top areas of medical spending is on high-cost imaging. The questions for specialists will be the following: What can we do to demonstrate the value of the care we deliver? What can we do to increase that value to our patient community? And how can that information be incorporated into a payment mechanism that pays specialists for the value they provide?

Sometimes, it's best to watch and wait instead of turning to expensive tests and high-cost imaging modalities such as CT scans or MRI scans. Doctors often practice defensive medicine, because they're afraid that if something is missed, the medico-legal consequences will be drastic. These lawsuits can be huge, and doctors are afraid that if they are sued for many millions of dollars, they'll be on the front page of the *New York Times*. It's easier for us to cover our butts and order imaging studies.

We know in our hearts they won't show anything, and it costs a doctor nothing to order those studies. However, it's going to cost the system tens of thousands of dollars, and it's going to be potentially invasive and unpleasant for the patient. We have to find ways to insure doctors for performing what's called "watchful waiting" instead of ordering up tests for fear of the legal ramifications of failing to do so.

You could say this is the next important area for the CCOs to work on: controlling costs associated with expensive aspects of medicine, where spending the money doesn't necessarily produce better results.

Mammography is one such area. This is a type of x-ray screening test performed to detect breast cancer early. In mammography, the question comes down to what's called a *callback rate*: If the doctor sees something concerning on a screening mammogram, then he needs to call the person back and do some additional imaging and diagnostic workups. In the United States the generally accepted, appropriate callback rate is less than 10 percent. That means that if the physician calls back a lot more than that—a rate, say of around 30 to 40 percent—that doctor is generating a lot of cost, exposing a lot of women to additional radiation, and unnecessarily creating a lot of unfounded emotional stress and anxiety.

Thus, the question becomes how we can incentivize radiologists to keep their screening rate to 10 percent? Can we pay them less if their callback rate goes up to the 20 to 30 percent range? This is the kind of issue that a CCO can explore. There are plenty of others, but this gives you a fair idea of the sorts of things we think about.

In short, it's perfectly understandable that doctors would resist a change, especially one that has any sort of government mandate attached to it. That's just not what doctors like, and there's so much fear right now in the medical community about the ability of doctors just to survive economically going forward. The good news is that, once people see how the CCOs enable them to serve more people—and serve them more efficiently and more effectively, without a loss in income—they generally sign on. It might not happen immediately, but the trend is certainly pointing to our approach to medicine as a better way to go.

CHAPTER 8:

HOW THE AFFORDABLE CARE ACT CHANGED EVERYTHING

With the passage of the Affordable Care Act, our Medicaid population in Yamhill County basically doubled. Initially, we'd had about twelve thousand members in our CCO. The relaxed income requirements of the Affordable Care Act pushed out the qualifications for coverage to 138 percent of the federal poverty level. As a result, we saw Medicaid membership increase to between twenty-four thousand and twenty-five thousand covered lives. You can imagine the kind of change this meant for an entity that had only been in existence for less than a year.

Once we knew that the ACA was coming, we held many conversations on the topic. We tried to strategize about how to serve this large influx of folks. We worked closely with the primary care providers to determine the number of new members they could accept. We called around and did surveys, and then created a procedure to assign members based on their location in the county. We also spent a great deal of time discussing the already pent-up demand for medical services for people who had previously not been served.

Now, it's not as though these people who now qualified for Medicaid had just moved to Yamhill County. Many of them might have had Medicaid in the past, or perhaps they had been employed and had commercial insurance. But for one reason or another, at this point in their lives, they'd lacked coverage for some meaningful period, and they were part of this expansion of our Medicaid population.

It was incredibly difficult for us to determine what type of care they were currently receiving, if any. Did they have a regular primary care provider? How often did they go to the emergency department? Was there a lingering health issue, such as addiction or a mental health problem, or was there a need for a larger procedure, such as a joint replacement or back surgery? We simply lacked the data that would allow us to predict what this population would be presenting once they received coverage.

We weren't entirely in the dark, however. Some data suggested that more than half of these folks had a diagnosed behavioral health problem for which they were not receiving treatment. Other data suggested that up to 25 percent of these individuals had diabetes, and in most cases, the condition was poorly managed. Thus, we did have a few data points to inform us about this population, but for the most part, our vision was limited.

Our approach was to make sure that our primary care providers were supported, both through the payment they received for healthcare and through additional funding of team-based care, so that they could hire enough behaviorists to take on the additional responsibilities these new members would require.

Whatever medical care patients had sought in the past was probably intermittent and ad hoc. They might have been seen in the emergency department, but they most certainly were not involved in a patient-centered primary care home. We expected that they would have lacked access to care and certainly had little access to preventative health services. Our strategy was to ensure that our primary care clinics and patient centered primary care homes would be ready to receive these folks and serve them.

The great influx of patients due to the Affordable Care Act demonstrated a new value of having a community-governed healthcare model. Instead of trying to create alliances to serve them, or simply serve them in the siloed fashion of the past, our planning sessions included hospital administrative leadership, specialists, and primary care providers from the physician community, as well as members of the dental care community and leadership from the behavioral health community.

We all knew each other because we had been working together as part of the CCO. Because we were all at the table together, and because we had these prior relationships, we could now have extremely open discussions about challenging issues like funding. We were able to acknowledge, as a community, that primary care had been dramatically underfunded for many years.

It was extremely helpful for everyone present to hear the leadership from primary care clinics speaking about the struggles they had in hiring and paying for staff and paying for medical supplies. There was concern, early on, that there might be backlash in some parts of the community—hospitals and specialists, most notably—when it came to paying more for primary care providers. Yet, the CCO system had demonstrated clearly to all of us that primary care providers were truly the cornerstone of our healthcare delivery system. With that in mind, we knew we needed to support them with more funding.

Remarkably, the group developed a comfort level with the idea of paying the primary care providers more, since they were indeed the front lines of serving the Medicaid community. Because we were all at the table and all of us had seen and acknowledged the problem, we were all able to come together and support the concept of higher payment for primary health providers.

Funding wasn't the only issue, however. We also had some physicians who had completed their training twenty, or even thirty, years ago. They had become quite comfortable with the status quo in managing their practices. So here we were, with a CCO trying to encourage them to do all sorts of different things like team-based care and paying for metrics. For these doctors, it was a whole new way of doing business, and the change was not a comfortable one. The analogy I liked to use was that we were trying to rebuild an airplane while it was flying.

The primary care clinics were now packed every day, seeing lots of people. At the same time, the CCOs were trying to work with these overstressed healthcare environments and get them to add on services and measure their performance in different ways than they had in the past. It was a struggle at first, and although most of our providers eventually embraced and supported the CCO approach, some skepticism remains. It still takes a lot of work and time to teach individuals what we are trying to do.

These challenges were certainly exacerbated by the doubling of our Medicaid community with the Affordable Care Act—but at the same time, we now had the opportunity to serve more people, which, of course, we embraced.

It's not as though these primary care providers had been operating well below capacity. Their patient levels had leapt up because of the new legislation. So, getting them to do new things and apply new metrics while trying to manage a vastly increased patient load was not easy.

The state of Oregon pitched in. The Oregon Health Authority—which, as I mentioned, oversees the CCOs—approved additional funding to be used as "transformation funds." The Yamhill County CCO received around $2 million to fund transformation programs such as supporting behaviorists for primary care clinics and other programs that would help build out our team-based approach to care. But now we had to come up with a way to distribute those funds to the community.

We did it as a collaborative grant-review process. We came up with an application and then I worked with different clinics and community organizations, in my role as a health strategy officer, to develop programs that would improve care and help us meet some of our metrics.

For example, we worked closely with one of our local hospitals on the development of an emergency-department observation unit. The idea behind the unit was simple.

Sometimes, when people come to the emergency department, they're ill and they may not be completely stable—but they're not sick enough to admit to the hospital. At the same time, the ED doc is uncomfortable discharging them.

One of the conditions that might trigger this situation is kidney stones. Perhaps the patient has pain and some blood in his urine, and the doctors cannot be sure if the stone will pass. If they could just give him some pain medication to get him comfortable, and provide him with a lot of hydration, that would help push the stone out.

Folks like these aren't quite ready to go home, but to admit them for a hospital course is a bit much. Today, there's a growing trend to place these patients in a third category instead of either discharging them or admitting them. This third category is called observational status, which allows them to come to the hospital for a limited period—up to forty-eight hours—and simply be observed. That observation would take place under the guidance of an emergency doctor, so the patient would not have to be admitted or seen by a specialist and, therefore, incur a whole new set of charges.

We were able to work with the emergency department of one of our local hospitals to fund the development of an ED observation program, so that they could develop this model of care. Without our funding, they would have been limited in their ability to pay for the staff time to get the program running.

The new ED observation program witnessed a decrease in the number of folks admitted to the hospital, and patient satisfaction has increased. That's because these individuals realize they don't need to be admitted to the hospital and seen by a whole group of doctors, which can be intimidating. Now they could simply be observed for a longer period.

The Affordable Care Act has been advantageous for the provision of medical care to low-income Americans. Prior to the ACA, we had uninsured rates in Yamhill County of up to 25 percent of our population. Because these individuals lacked regular access to primary care, they would go to the emergency department whenever they needed medical help—and of course, that's the most expensive form of care there is.

Because ED doctors usually don't know patients coming into their departments, they take a very conservative approach to treating individuals who lack insurance. They will do a lot of medical tests, including imaging tests. The care they deliver is very expensive and, quite frankly, sometimes it's "over the top," but you can understand where they're coming from; they don't want to take a chance on missing something with a patient they've never seen before.

So, we really experienced the worst of both worlds. Individuals who lacked insurance went to an emergency department where they weren't getting the appropriate level of care, and from a financial standpoint, they were getting the most expensive care imaginable. They would also have to go through the discomfort (for them) and the expense (for us) of CT scans, ultrasounds, and MRIs that weren't necessarily indicated.

The doctors might also be thinking that, since these folks don't have insurance or might be homeless, the medical care might never get paid for. Much of the work we were all doing, prior to the Affordable Care Act, was essentially charity care.

Now, most of these individuals have insurance and we can bill on Medicaid. Granted, we aren't getting the same rates for them that we would get for commercially insured patients, but at least it was something. In my radiology practice, bad debt has decreased dramatically, to the point where it's 80 percent below what it was prior to the passage of the ACA. The benefits are manifold.

First, the patients are getting appropriate care in appropriate settings. The ED doctors are most likely happier, because when these patients present at the emergency department, they can see whether they have insurance through the Yamhill CCO. They can look up their primary care provider and arrange for follow-up care after these folks have been seen in the emergency department. Prior to the ACA, these individuals would not have had regular, assigned primary-care providers, and they would have had limited access—or even no access—to follow-up care, because they simply didn't have anywhere to go.

It almost certainly creates a sense of relief for the emergency department doctors to now know that someone out there can take ownership of the patient. The patients are happier, too, because they know exactly where their clinic is and who their doctor is; that information is all on the back of their insurance card. In the past, they often didn't know where to go or whom to call if they got sick, so they had to go to the emergency department. Often, they would arrive confused and frustrated because their only option was to seek emergency care.

People are concerned about the cost of fulfilling on the Affordable Care Act, but I see many benefits to payers. We can now start to develop and collect data on these folks. We can measure their medical-use history and begin to forecast what costs they may incur going forward and what kinds of services they might need. This allows us to budget better.

Prior to the ACA, when the income requirements were lower, it was very difficult to get a handle on the needs of this population. One month, they might be covered by Medicaid, and another month, they might not be. This is a concept called the "churn," describing individuals who "churn" in and out of Medicaid. It may well be that, during the month when they're not covered by Medicaid, they develop health problems that never get addressed. Then they stop working and their income dips, so they would qualify for Medicaid again—but now they've got all these new health problems and issues that are uncontrolled. That pushes costs higher. If only they could have stayed covered the entire time and had regular access to care, their conditions would have been better managed and would not have gotten out of control or been so expensive. Churn still happens, but to a lesser degree with the current model.

Many politicians love to bash the ACA and call it socialized medicine or an unfunded taxpayer liability or a blank check. Frankly, you can call it whatever you want, but the reality on the ground is that more people are getting more appropriate care than in the past. I'd like to invite anyone inveighing against the Affordable Care Act to come here to Oregon, talk to our doctors, talk to our hospitals, talk to our behaviorists, and talk to our patients. Then look at our numbers and discover that what I've been saying in this chapter is true. We're delivering better and more appropriate care to more people for less money.

CHAPTER 9:

BEHAVIORAL HEALTH IMPACTS PHYSICAL HEALTH,

SO WHY ARE WE IGNORING IT?

As we discussed earlier, the determinants of our health are not always what we think them to be. In fact, only about 20 percent of our actual health is impacted by the medical care we receive. This includes routine health screening exams; vaccines for infectious diseases like measles, mumps, or rubella; and prescriptions when we get sick. A much larger part of our health is a function of other things—the sorts of choices we make and the surroundings in which we live, all of which are removed from our traditional relationship with our doctor.

Let's look at that other 80 percent. The exact percentages in each of the following vary, depending on what research you read, but I think these are good summations.

The physical environment influences about 10 percent of our health. Some people have secure, stable housing, while others are homeless. Another important determinant is socioeconomic factors: our level of education; whether we have stable employment; whether we live in a safe, stable community; and whether we have a good family and social support network.

Another 30 percent of our health is affected by our behaviors and the choices we make. Do we use tobacco? Do we diet and exercise appropriately? Do we moderate and control our alcohol intake? Where are we with unsafe behaviors— anything from driving without a seatbelt to having unsafe sex to gambling uncontrollably, to the point where we are in debt? All these issues result in socioeconomic problems, and they can cause physical problems as well. So, you can see that the overwhelming majority of the factors regarding our health are the sorts of things that lie outside the traditional conversations between doctor and patient in an examination room.

Of course, there has been some overlap in which doctors address traditional behavioral health issues. Doctors may screen for depression, anxiety, and alcohol abuse. When they reflect on what they learned in medical school, however, they studied, for the most part, the organic components of the body: anatomy, physiology, biochemistry, histology, and pathology. Very little formal training is offered in terms of dealing with an individual's *behavioral* health. That's simply not a focus of traditional medical education for physicians, physician assistants, or nurse practitioners. They're all much more involved with what we traditionally think of when we consider medicine: treating the *physical* body.

If we step back and take a broader view, to be a healthcare provider means that we need to provide care in all determinants of health—not just the physical realm, but also the behavioral realm, as well as the socioeconomic and physical environment in which the patient lives. But are we really doing that?

Physicians might argue that they do have some behavioral health training. In my instance, I did a six-week rotation in psychiatry while I was in medical school. That, however, was the extent of the formal training I received in non-physical health issues. Yet, when individuals present to their doctor, their issues are often rooted in the behaviors they have chosen to pursue.

We are talking about obesity, diabetes, or high blood pressure, which are "lifestyle diseases." Maybe some people do make behavioral choices that affect their health—like stopping for a milkshake and fries on the way home from work or smoking in the car to cope with a long commute. From a medical standpoint, those so-called lifestyle diseases are within the physician's wheelhouse.

Often, physicians become frustrated with their patients. They're trying to help people lose weight, or trying to get them to take their high-blood-pressure medications, but people won't make those lifestyle choices. The problem is exacerbated for our Medicaid population, who come from the most disadvantaged sectors of our society. Working with low-income patients on their personal healthcare responsibilities is considerably harder than trying to get a middle-class person to quit the McDonald's drive-through on the way home from work.

Many of our Medicaid members have a history of physical abuse or sexual abuse. They've been through trauma. They suffer from addictions. They come from very hard backgrounds. Many have parents who immigrated here from another country, perhaps illegally. Since they were undocumented, the home in which they grew up was tenuous and unstable. Now, that upbringing results in the choices these individuals make and affects the behavioral- and physical-health resiliency they possess. This is not open to debate; this is a fact of life.

A physician or community of providers who just sits there and remains frustrated about Medicaid patients not taking their medications or not walking enough simply is not getting at the root of the problem.

The doctor may say, "I really didn't go into medicine to handle this. I wanted to diagnose and treat disease, and write prescriptions. But now I have to work in an environment where people just don't comply, and it's frustrating. What's the point?"

When our CCO here in Yamhill opened, the primary care doctors wanted to help our organization. They wanted to open their doors to see Medicaid members. At the same time, they were concerned that they would be overwhelmed by the behavioral health aspects that a lot of these patients would bring with them. The doctors were concerned that they might not be able to handle it all and actually help these people.

To address this critical concern, we elected to support a model of behavioral health integration, so that the funding of CCOs would take place under one global budget. From that budget, funding would pay for both physical health and behavioral health services. At the state level, it had always been the intention that behavioral and physical health would go hand in hand. They would work together toward the same mission and vision, under the same budget, and use the same set of metrics to measure performance and ultimately pay for that performance.

On the local level, it became the responsibility of the CCOs to take that mandate and operationalize it. Now, this sounds like a great idea. Let's integrate behavioral and physical health. Let's allow them to work together. But what would that look like, and then how do we use that idea to address the concerns of the primary care provider? How do we actually deal with the behavioral health issues of those members coming into our clinics?

One key was hiring what are called "behaviorists"— professionally trained psychologists who work within primary care clinics, side by side with the physicians.

Now, it's true that there's lots of waste in medicine. This is something that all doctors see, almost all the time. One of the subtler forms of waste is when an individual's skills aren't fully taken advantage of. In other words, an individual may have a certain level of training, but the job that person has only calls for them to use, say, half of the training.

For example, I was trained as a radiologist. I went to medical school for four years after college, and then went through six years of training—including an internship, residency, and fellowship training—so that I could learn how to interpret imaging exams. A lot of my time is invested—and a lot of society's time and resources are invested—in interpreting and dictating films, which makes my time relatively valuable.

Yet, sometimes, I'll spend fifteen minutes just trying to find a phone number and get a doctor on the phone to discuss an issue. In a perfect world, I would have someone helping me make that connection, or there would be a technological solution to make the connection for me. That's a simple example to show that there's a lot of waste within medicine. It's not all about overpaying for supplies. Sometimes, it is a waste of time and training that we really need to address.

If you're a physician, you should be diagnosing and treating; you shouldn't be trying to make phone calls or send e-mails and faxes or complete paperwork, tasks that are not actually appropriate for someone with your skill set. In the team-based approach to healthcare in our primary care clinics, one of the goals is to avoid having people do things that don't relate specifically to their unique ability and training. If we have people filling all the gaps, then everyone gets to do what he or she has been trained to do—what he or she went into medicine in the first place to accomplish.

How does this play out in reality? A physician might be part of a team in a primary care clinic, and he may have some behavioral training. Yet he may not be the best person to counsel a woman who has just suffered a first-trimester miscarriage. Let's say the patient is a teen. She was pregnant, but today's ultrasound indicates that she's lost the baby. She's going to be emotionally upset.

A physician can address the physical diagnosis and the symptoms she may experience. But in an optimized clinic, that same physician probably is not the best person to help the teen work through the emotions she will have and help her deal with the loss, the suffering, and the grieving that she's going through. Of course, the physician has a role in this process— but there are other professionals better-trained to help with this aspect of treatment who can dedicate the time to deliver the care this patient needs.

If there were a behaviorist in that clinic, the behaviorist would be much better-equipped than the doctor, typically, to handle that situation. The behaviorist would have a much better skill set in this area and probably would have experience with these situations. Behaviorists also are licensed to provide these higher-level behavioral health and counseling services.

In a behavioral-integration healthcare model, the physician might see the patient with the miscarriage and make the diagnosis and discuss her physical health treatment. But then that doctor calls in the behaviorist, who happens to be in the same clinic. The doctor does what we call a "warm handoff," which just means having the behaviorist come in and see the patient during the same visit. The behaviorist now can talk about grief and loss, and provide some empathy and comfort, which the physician isn't as well-qualified to do, because that's not the "top of his license." But this *is* the top of the behaviorist's license.

You could almost think of it as a preemptive strike—to help the patient avoid issues like depression or relationship concerns that would arise if they did not receive immediate attention. A teen pregnancy resulting in a miscarriage is a set-up for depression, or perhaps the young woman is engaged in a relationship in which she didn't have a choice about becoming pregnant. Maybe she's being manipulated in some way, so she's unable to use contraception and prevent an unwanted pregnancy. The behaviorist can work with the patient and get to the root of the problem.

For this patient, we can deal with the acute problem of the suffering that attends a miscarriage, but more importantly, the behaviorist can discuss the issue of why she became pregnant in the first place. What led to the pregnancy? Does the patient have safe and stable housing, or was this a case of abuse? What behavioral issues need to be considered to prevent this from happening again in the future?

These conversations take time and skill, and, in these areas, behaviorists are simply more adept than a physician who is trained to offer a diagnosis. Perhaps it sounds a little idealistic, but this sort of intervention might just prevent a future unwanted teen pregnancy and, therefore, it might prevent another unwanted miscarriage.

Things can work in the other direction as well. Integration also means putting physicians into behavioral health clinics, which is something we've been able to do through the CCOs. Often, individuals in our system only receive care from their behavioral provider. Maybe they haven't been able to engage a primary care provider for one reason or another. They may not have any physical health problems, or perhaps they do, but they just could never get in to see a doctor. Some psychiatric medications they take might have a negative effect on their bodies. Antipsychotics, for example, can result in weight gain or even obesity, and that creates its own set of problems.

We've been able to begin to put primary-care providers into behavioral health clinics. Now, if someone goes to see their counselor and their medication regimen is making them feel poorly, or causing weight gain that is resulting in health problems, there's a doctor right there who can address those specific issues. That doctor can test and screen for diabetes or see if the patient has high cholesterol. If the patient's primary relationship is with a behavioral care provider, why shouldn't there be a doctor on the scene? That way, we can make that warm handoff from behaviorist to physician, if such a handoff is indicated.

As an aside, doctors have become much more open to the idea of behavioral health in recent decades. When I first began to learn about healthcare transformation, I was part of a cohort of Oregonians who went up to Anchorage, Alaska, for a four-day visit to a healthcare system called the Southcentral Foundation. It's a Native American–run healthcare system that arose in response to the need to provide better healthcare for Native Americans back in the 1970s.

Back then, folks felt that if they were going to the hospital, they were going there to die. They did not feel as though they were being cared for in the hospital. In the '70s, these services were administered, funded, and run by the federal government, with little autonomy given to Native American populations. Federal legislation was eventually passed which changed this. It gave controlling governance of the healthcare system to Native Americans. In Alaska, this led to the establishment of the Southcentral Foundation.

Some of the changes they were able to implement were things that the federal government would never have come up with in a million years. For instance, the physical buildings where their medical care was delivered were imposing and intimidating. Many of these Native Americans lived in structures made from natural materials, and they lived in remote and rural places. When they would go to a city hospital, they would find themselves in a concrete-and-steel building with glass and florescent lights. It was very uninviting. They didn't want to go, and when they did go, the care they received came from individuals who were not fellow Native Americans. The communication was different. The way they were treated was not particularly appropriate, so they weren't getting the care they needed and deserved.

Over the past forty years, however, medical care for Native Americans in Alaska has undergone a huge transformation. They have done amazing things in building new facilities that have a Native American feel to them.

For example, when you go into the large outpatient clinic building in Anchorage, on the first floor, you will find no typical, Western-style "medical clinics." Instead, you will find a garden with different herbs and plants that Native Americans use for natural healing and a healing-arts center with a traditional healer on staff. Thus, the building doesn't have a medical feel. It doesn't smell like a clinic or hospital when you walk inside, so you don't feel as though you're going to get poked and prodded. It's a much more welcoming, warm environment.

In Anchorage, the realization came early that a team-based approach, integrating behavioral healthcare along with traditional medical care, was very important. The marriage of behavioral and traditional healthcare that we witnessed in Anchorage was highly influential in terms of what we created here in Oregon.

In the facility in Anchorage, you will see "talking rooms"—places where patients and healthcare providers, and perhaps a family member or other member of the care team, can sit down and talk about issues that may be impacting the patient's health. There's no exam table, no stethoscope on the wall, and no cotton balls in the glass container (for what purpose, no one ever seems to know). There's no medical aspect to the environment in that room. It's just a place where you can go to discuss behavioral, socioeconomic, or physical determinants of health—without having to feel as though you're in the medical realm.

In Yamhill, we don't have talking rooms yet, but I'm hoping that we will soon. We want to talk about people's behavioral health, and we need to do it in a non-medically threatening environment, where people don't feel as though a rushed doctor with a white coat and stethoscope just wants to poke and prod them. Imagine how different it would be if we could provide a comfortable room with nice chairs in which people could sit in a relaxed fashion and talk with providers who really want to listen. Maybe that's a better way to start addressing health issues that aren't necessarily medically related.

A conversation in a talking room might begin with the patient explaining that she's depressed. Traditionally, we would provide antidepressant medication, and that would be that. Now, however, we could attempt to determine why the patient is depressed. Maybe she doesn't have access to reliable transportation and she can never get to her job on time. So, she loses her job, she gets more depressed, she loses her health insurance because she's not working, and then she can never get in to see a doctor. Then the depression gets worse, so she starts overeating, smoking, or drinking, and starts on a downward spiral.

Maybe all she needs is a social worker to help her with transportation so she can get to her job on time. The talking room is a place where we could identify that need. We could then bring in the social worker to help with transportation issues or bring in the behaviorist to talk about any behavioral health-related issues from which the patient was suffering. One conversation could save thousands of dollars in inappropriate medical care that doesn't get to the heart of the issue. More to the point, one conversation like that, with the appropriate integrated team members present and solving the problem, could save a life.

As I said, we don't have talking rooms yet, but I hope we will soon. In the meantime, the model for integrating behavioral care along with medical care is something that arose from that trip to Anchorage. The Southcentral Foundation, you could say, was the place where the light bulb went on for us.

They had one integrated healthcare system. We did not. We had independent clinics, some clinics that were for-profit corporations, some hospitals that were for-profit corporations, and a large, Catholic hospital system.

We recognized from the start that it would not be easy to implement any sort of broad, sweeping change. My initial role was to share the ideas we had and talk about the success they were enjoying in Alaska, and try to encourage people to adopt aspects of it. Thus, in part, the behaviorist program has taken root not just in Yamhill, but also in many of the CCOs across the state of Oregon.

The finances for this process are still evolving. Behaviorists can bill for many of their services, but not all of them. This gets back to the whole idea of flexible spending. Sometimes a bus pass or an air conditioner can achieve so much more than a medical prescription.

I mentioned earlier that the former governor would often tell the story about the poor, old woman with congestive heart failure who got sick every summer because she lived in a walk-up apartment with oppressive heat. She would become dehydrated and this would lead to congestive heart failure. In the past, her monthly visits to the emergency department would cost tens of thousands of dollars.

If we could just buy this patient an air conditioner for $150 to keep her apartment cool, she wouldn't become dehydrated and go into congestive heart failure. We could save tons of money. But if we were going to be able to buy that air conditioner, we needed to be able to use medical dollars in a flexible way, and pay for things that aren't traditionally considered medical-care services.

That story leads to the question of how we fund the behaviorists. We use a component of our funds to pay for their services with what's called "flexible funding." We simply designate their services as health-related and pay for them directly out of our global budget.

Our challenge now is to tie their work into some sort of measurable return on investment. That takes time. Since we're still early on in this process of healthcare transformation, we don't have a lot of experience to draw upon as to how to make those connections between spending money and getting results. It's not as though there are a lot of software platforms that do it easily! We're evolving in terms of how we tie the work of behaviorists to actual decreases in cost.

We are seeing an increase in patient satisfaction on surveys at clinics with behaviorists. We can also objectively track results with certain individuals, like the teen mother who underwent the miscarriage.

Where does it go from here? We must be cautious with the way we use our flexible-spending dollars. We must track how the money is spent to make sure that it's not wasted, and that we're really getting better outcomes—decreased costs and lower mortality and morbidity eventually.

When you consider the fact that 80 percent of our health is a function of the things that occur in our lives outside the doctor's office, it's clear we need to focus on that 80 percent. And our experience here in Yamhill is that, when we do, we get better outcomes.

CHAPTER 10:

BOOTS ON THE GROUND:

THE COMMUNITY PARAMEDICINE PROGRAM

A unique aspect of Yamhill County is our highly-sophisticated wine industry. As a result, it's not uncommon to see a Ferrari or a high-powered Audi tooling around the area. At the same time, we are an isolated place where much of the county is served by the kind of dirt-and-gravel roads those Ferraris and Audis will never see.

At the end of those roads, you might find a thirty- or forty-year-old mobile home, its condition poor, lacking electricity, or even running water. The folks who live in these mobile homes may have no transportation. They're living very isolated lives. We have some rudimentary public transportation in the county, but it doesn't cover everyone. Since these individuals cannot easily get into town, they can't seek basic services, like treatment from a primary care physician.

The transportation barrier is severe. Sometimes, it's because these folks lack a car of their own, or there's only one car and the breadwinner works, so the car is not available to the spouse. Perhaps they don't have a car at all, for economic reasons, or perhaps they've had one or more DUIs and cannot drive. Consequently, regular medical attention, especially preventative care, doesn't become a priority until a health situation becomes an emergency. When things turn into an emergency, their only option is to call 911 and have an ambulance come and bring them to the hospital.

Let's say one of these folks gets sick. Maybe she can't breathe. Maybe she's running a high fever, or sleep, for whatever reason, is eluding her. Calling 911 and getting an ambulance really is the best medical decision she can make for herself or her loved ones, since she has no other options. It's easy for people who have regular access to medical care (whether we have Ferraris or not) to criticize these folks and say that they don't need to call an ambulance if they only have a cough. But if you've had a cough for two weeks and no car, and you can't get in to see a primary care doctor—well then, yes, perhaps you do need to call an ambulance.

Transportation is a huge issue in Yamhill County and many other rural areas. We all know that crisis and opportunity are covered by the same Chinese symbol. This healthcare crisis became an opportunity when the West Valley Fire Department saw this as a chance to serve in a new and, we think, exciting way.

Not only are many of the people in western, rural Yamhill County isolated geographically and lacking in transportation, but they're also very independent. They don't ask for help, and they're skeptical when people come into their lives trying to offer help. In some instances, isolation is a way of life these people have chosen. For others, it's just something they were born into or had thrust upon them. Learning who these people are and what their needs are can be challenging, since they're not actively reaching out for help. In many cases, it isn't until they visit the emergency room that we even hear about them.

The West Valley Fire Department, which serves the most rural areas in our county, realized that there were many people who were essentially living in the shadows. These are the folks who would be taken by ambulance from their homes to the emergency department, either once or twice a week or several times a year. Perhaps these individuals have asthma that's not well-controlled—or they can't manage their medication, or they smoke, or perhaps they live in a house with a wood-burning stove. Maybe they have diabetes that they cannot control because they do not have access to medication. These are the folks who are always calling 911, during their frequent, acute exacerbations of chronic conditions, which they do not necessarily manage well.

The West Valley Fire Department realized that there had to be a better way to treat these folks, and this led to the creation of our Community Paramedicine Program. When you think about it, the paramedics and ambulance drivers are the individuals in our healthcare system who already have a relationship with the rural individuals I'm talking about here. These folks trust their paramedics and ambulance drivers. They know them. They know that, when they call 911, these people will come and bring them to the emergency department to get the treatment they need. The paramedics know where these people live. They're familiar with the backcountry roads. Often, they live in these communities, so they know what types of issues are going on.

The West Valley Fire Department decided it wanted to start a Community Paramedicine Program. We had a grant process through the Yamhill CCO called Transform Forward. This is funding from the state of Oregon to allow CCOs to fund novel healthcare-delivery systems, approaches that would innovate and transform the way care is provided. The West Valley Fire Department put forth a grant application, and we gave them some startup money, so that they could buy a vehicle and do some staff training. We then contracted with them, on a long-term basis, to pay them to perform a certain number of visits a month to these otherwise isolated individuals.

One of the types of services they perform is to visit individuals identified as "high utilizers" of emergency-department services. We'll send someone in the local community to reach out to the folks and actually go to their homes, to see why these individuals keep coming to the emergency department. Is there some sort of issue in their physical environment? Maybe it's that wood-burning stove. Maybe it's someone else smoking in the house. Maybe it's the lack of transportation I mentioned. These providers now visit these individuals to perform in-home safety checks. While they're visiting, they also look at their medications and help them get organized, as I discussed earlier.

The patients are already familiar with the drivers, because they've been seeing that ambulance show up month after month. Thus, when the ambulance driver comes by, along with the paramedic, the patients are comfortable with these visits. It costs considerably less to visit a person and check on him or her in a non-emergent fashion, and there's also much less pressure and drama involved.

By funding this model, the CCO can have paramedics working with these people when their asthma, diabetes, or other conditions are not in an acute phase. This way, the paramedic has the luxury of time to ask, "Well, what's triggering these exacerbations? Is it the meds? Is it the wood-burning stove? What is it?" Now they can go out there, work with the person, and see what might be triggering that asthma or other condition.

We see that these individuals become part of the healthcare system in a new way. Our hospitals are under a mandate to limit the number of patients who are readmitted or come back to the hospital in thirty days. If a greater-than-acceptable number of patients are readmitted within thirty days, the hospital can lose payments from both Medicare and Medicaid. Thus, hospitals are highly motivated and incentivized to make sure that when individuals are discharged, they don't come back right away. Because of the Community Paramedicine Program, we now have individuals living in better situations at home, which means that there are fewer readmissions. In short, everybody wins.

The hospitals have contracted with this new Community Paramedicine Program to enable home visits two to three days after the patient is discharged. If that patient is identified as being at high risk for readmission, the paramedic goes out and checks up on him to see if he understands all his discharge instructions and see if he's able to schedule with a primary care provider for a routine follow-up after discharge. If necessary, the paramedic can even take samples for lab tests.

In the past, an individual with transportation issues would never have been able to experience these services. He or she likely would be ticketed for a quick readmission to the emergency department with no long-term benefit to his or her healthcare. Simply not having labs re-checked increases the risk of readmission. You can see how the totality of this approach—proactive visits, and then post-hospital-admission visits—changes the equation for the patients, the hospitals, and the CCO as a whole.

Complicating matters, some of the roads in the western part of our county are steep, mountainous, and winding. Some are in poor condition, with small, one-lane bridges. Others are prone to being closed due to weather, flooding from a creek, a landslide, or a fallen tree. As the crow flies, we're talking about thirty miles, but the country can be quite rugged and remote.

Yamhill County, thanks to our intrepid West Valley Fire Department, was one of the first CCOs to put dollars behind a Community Paramedicine Program. The hospital is now paying for the program to see Medicare patients as well as some commercially insured patients. This is yet another example of how the CCOs, which were created to serve the Medicaid community, have had what you call a ripple effect across all healthcare providers. This program benefits the entire population, beyond just the Medicaid folks. Hospitals now are financially at risk for readmissions of all kinds, whether we are talking about Medicaid, Medicare, or commercially insured patients. It's easy to see how a program that began under the auspices of the CCO has ramifications for all of us.

It would be premature to discuss the overall financial effect this one program has had on Yamhill County's Medicaid spending, but it's fair to say that every readmission we prevent with a home visit saves us between $10,000 and $15,000. This program currently serves only a small part of the western area of the county, and we are avoiding five or six readmissions a month. So, we're already talking about a savings of $50,000 to $90,000 a month, with just a small part of our county being addressed. As the program grows, so will those numbers.

Keep in mind that this is a new way to serve folks. We are creating a lot of new positions, from the paramedics we've discussed here to community health workers to behaviorists. We're also evolving new requirements for continuing education. The financial returns on investment look promising, indeed.

On top of that, it's just satisfying to know that we are creating a substantial, long-lasting improvement in the health care of many folks who live so far from our primary care homes that they have never had access to this level of medical care before. We can intervene meaningfully, instead of in repeated ways that don't have a long-term payoff, and we're able to do so in a way that preserves their dignity while we're improving their health.

CHAPTER 11:

FLEXIBLE FUNDS:

PAYING FOR NONTRADITIONAL MEDICAL GOODS AND SERVICES

O ne of the most exciting aspects of healthcare reform is paying for healthcare goods and services in nontraditional ways. Traditionally, the only way you get paid for providing a healthcare good or service is by use of a CPT code—essentially, a billing code. If there's no billing code attached to what you're doing, then the third-party payer does not have to pay for it.

The challenge is that many goods and services that could help our overall delivery of health care don't have billing codes attached. That's because, as we've discussed throughout the book, much of our health is determined by what happens outside the four walls of a medical clinic. Only 20 percent of our health is the result of what happens inside clinics or because of medical care. CPT codes abound for those goods and services. But how do we pay for things that affect the other 80 percent of our health?

At first glance, it makes no sense that a healthcare payer should be required to pay for only 20 percent of the healthcare of the folks he ostensibly serves. Housing, employment, and other socioeconomic factors are critically important when it comes to our health. Thus, the question becomes this: how do we redirect healthcare spending so that we can assist people in these areas that are so vital to their wellness?

The Oregon state legislation enabling the Coordinated Care Model gave communities something of a blank slate to figure out how to provide new ways of funding for these new categories of spending, many of which have never been considered traditional healthcare expenditures in the past. The term used is "flexible services" and refers to offerings on which CCO's have the flexibility to spend funds. How can you use the money you receive from the state to pay for healthcare and pay for things that do not have CPT codes attached to them? Flexible services *is* the Oregon approach.

Certainly government, both state and federal, has spent money on housing and employment for individuals in the past, and they have also authorized spending for behavioral health. However, using flexible funding in the medical realm to address social issues has seldom been tried before.

It all goes back to that classic story about the low-income woman, living in the second-floor apartment, who needed the air conditioner. As I've mentioned, she's eighty years old, it's ninety degrees out, and she's sitting in her apartment sweating and becoming dehydrated. Her heart is working harder and harder to keep up with her fluid and electrolyte imbalances. Before long, her heart cannot keep up with the condition, and she ends up spending a very expensive week in the hospital.

That whole incident, and all the costs associated with it, could have been prevented if we could have just bought her an air conditioner. Unfortunately, there was no CPT code for an air conditioner and no place in the budget to pay for that sort of thing. Flexible funding means getting the community to buy air conditioners—to purchase the things that really impact our health, yet cannot be coded.

We've started down the flexible services path here in Yamhill County, but there's nothing easy about it. It's great to have a blank slate, because there are so many things you can buy to help people with their health. You can buy them fresh, nutritious foods in the form of a subscription to a community-supported agriculture program, through which they receive fresh vegetables delivered to their homes on a weekly basis. Or you can help them pay for rent in a more safe and hospitable environment. You can get them some job training so they can acquire skills to get a job with commercial health insurance, which means that eventually, they will be able to leave the ranks of Medicaid patients.

There is in fact so much opportunity to serve in this manner that the whole thing can be overwhelming for small communities like ours. Here in Yamhill, we're trying to start a new healthcare plan, and suddenly, we're able to purchase goods and services that in the past, we could never touch.

It all sounds great, but there's an inordinate amount of stress associated with this responsibility. We cannot pay for *all* these services for *all* of our folks; we would bust our budget. It's also difficult to know which of these services would provide great health outcomes. Where's the research? Along with the responsibility to our population, we also have a fiscal responsibility to the taxpayers and the state.

One positive aspect of CPT codes is related to the notion of practicing evidence-based medicine. Most of the goods and services paid for with CPT codes are backed by rigorous scientific studies demonstrating that they are beneficial. We don't have as much data indicating whether, from an economic standpoint, we're getting a solid return on investment in flexible services. But at least we know that various treatments do produce certain health outcomes.

For example, if someone breaks a bone, we know he'll get a better outcome if he gets a cast and sees an orthopedic surgeon. Cause and effect. But do people really get better health outcomes if you buy them a bike so they can cycle to work? Where's the data on that? Does the data indicate that everyone given a bike would use it? Or is there simply a subset of people who would actually use that bike and benefit from it? Should you buy them gym memberships instead?

The problem is that, without hard data, the whole thing can become fodder for those who are searching for "waste, fraud, and abuse" in every corner. If we don't spend the money properly, we not only have an economic or budget issue, we have a potential political problem as well. Our approach to flexible funding has focused on funding those goods and services that align with what we are already trying to do. And that brings us back to the question of metrics.

As we've discussed, one of the metrics by which CCOs are held accountable is performing adolescent well-child checks: making sure that adolescents come in every year for various screenings and appropriate immunizations. Are they meeting certain milestones as they grow? It's challenging to get kids to come to the doctor, however. They're busy and they're healthy. They ask, "Why do I need to go to the doctor? I don't have any problems."

So, we used some of our flexible services to support the purchase of gift cards from local bookstores as well as from Apple. Any child who came in for an adolescent well-child check—and overall health screening—would receive a gift card. There's no CPT code for a gift card to iTunes! Since we have this new flexibility, however, we can buy these gift cards and give them to clinics, thus incentivizing kids to come in and seek better health care.

From the standpoint of the organization, it's a win for us because, if the provider clinics get more of these young people in the door, then we can meet our financial-incentive metric as an organization. The dollars we spend on gift cards come back many times over in terms of the bonus dollars we receive, which we allocate to our primary-care clinics so they can hire more staff and improve the care they deliver. It's a virtuous cycle, a chain reaction of benefits that begins with spreading the news that, if you're a kid and you come in for a checkup, you'll get an iTunes or a bookstore gift card.

While gift cards to incentivize young people sounds simple enough, the complications arise when there are dollars to be spent and no traditional limitations on *how* they are to be spent. To put it simply, everyone has an opinion. We wanted to be careful to avoid creating infighting among our various constituents. We did not want to have the medical community fighting with the behavioral health community, and both of those groups fighting with the dental health community, to get at some of those dollars. We realized that we needed a policy around how those dollars would be distributed. What was the process? What dollar amounts would be attached?

We created a workgroup along with our physical health providers, behavioral health community, and dental health community. By working closely with them, we were able to create the language that addressed how flexible spending would take place. The policy the groups created was then approved by the board. This allows us to take the blank slate we were given and begin to build a structure around it.

Our work in this area is far from finished, but we have become more experienced as different requests come in. Again, when you have dollars to spend, you must have a process in place, because otherwise, there would be havoc.

One area that made sense from the start, in terms of flexible services, is our Persistent Pain Program, which educates people on what chronic pain is and how to deal with it in ways other than using opioids. We realized that this spending would support both physical health and behavioral health. It seemed appropriate to use some dollars to fund the building of a new clinic, as well as to pay for staff training.

Now, when a patient completes the program, we buy them a small gift to acknowledge their success—something that can also help them with their health on a long-term basis. Those gifts might include bicycles or yoga studio memberships. Once again, there is no CPT code for a yoga studio membership! Without the flexible services, we would never have had the dollars to pay for that sort of thing. You could say it's a nontraditional approach—but when you look at the opioid epidemic in every corner of the United States, we've got to find new ways to cope, because the alternative is unthinkable.

Prescription painkillers are a huge problem in the United States, along with the overdoses associated with those drugs. About sixteen thousand people die in the United States every year due to an overdose of prescription painkillers.[5] From what source do you get a prescription? You get it from your doctor or some other healthcare provider. This means that we doctors, unfortunately, are causing what you could call provider-promoted deaths. You can't really blame the providers, because some of these patients are getting drugs from multiple doctors. At the same time, you cannot deny that sixteen thousand people a year are dying from painkillers which they obtained from written prescriptions.

Another statistic that gives one pause is that, as recently as a few years ago, one in twenty people in the United States reported using prescription painkillers for nonmedical reasons.[6] Again, where are they getting these drugs? Not on the street, but rather, in their doctors' offices. They're getting them through prescriptions and this is a huge issue for society.

The challenge, as providers will tell you, "We're so busy, we don't have the resources. We can't address all these people's complex issues: the behavioral, medical, and addictive problems they have. We can't focus on all their determinants of health. They're in pain, so we give them painkillers." It sounds reasonable. We write the prescription and we're giving them what they want.

We're giving providers a different option from simply picking up the pen and writing a Vicodin prescription. Now they can pick up that same pen and give these folks a referral to our Persistent Pain Program. The evidence shows that opioids

---

5   http://www.cdc.gov/drugoverdose/data/overdose.html
6   http://www.cdc.gov/vitalsigns/painkilleroverdoses/

do a poor job of managing non-cancer chronic pain, but people with that sort of pain are the ones who are taking these opioids, getting addicted to them, and overdosing on them.

This is one of our bigger programs, because it's certainly one of our bigger problems. We actually built a physical space for a classroom, as well as a counseling area, so that these individuals can be cared for properly and effectively.

It's worth noting that the whole opioid addiction issue and the Persistent Pain Program were not created top down and then thrust on our community providers. Instead, this was a problem that our doctors in the community identified. It was not the state that identified this issue; it was the CCO itself, based on what the providers were coming in and saying. The power of the CCO is that providers are involved in its governance and have a real say in how the organization is run, how money is spent, and how new programs are developed.

Empowering healthcare providers sounds like a nice idea, but with the CCOs, it's a reality, and our program is successful because our doctors have a greater say than ever in healthcare spending in our county. We did not receive an outside mandate saying, "You need to start a pain program, and this is what it's going to look like." Instead, the program was developed internally when the providers said, "We need a pain program. This is what it should look like, this is what we should spend on it, and this is where it should be located."

It would have been terrific if an insurance company had said, "Hey, guys—here's a million bucks. Why don't you start a pain program?" But that's not how things happened. Instead, the providers bore the financial risk within the CCO when they said, "Let's take this money that belongs to our community and spend it on a program that we consider valuable." That's why community-governed healthcare plans like ours have the potential to be so successful—because the power is in the hands of the providers to determine how to serve, instead of the typical situation in which what they can do is mandated and limited from above.

Let's turn to another program that flexible services has allowed us to support: a Peer-Support Program. We have individuals in our community with conditions like diabetes, hypertension, or behavioral health issues. These folks have successfully learned how to address these conditions; they've learned skills for managing and coping with them. They know what the local resources are. We supported a Peer-Support Program to train and employ these folks to work with others in the community who have similar conditions.

Peer-to-peer support has turned out to be extremely valuable. Typically, if you have a medical problem, you go to your doctor and he prescribes some medicine and tells you when to follow up or where to go to get additional help. But the doctor does not live with this problem the way the patient does. The doctor does not know what it's like to be obese with high blood pressure and diabetes and live in Yamhill County. Maybe the doctor's fit and has no health problems, which means that, for all his training and good intentions, he may not be able to relate to the patient's problems.

Consequently, he may not be giving the patient the advice that's really needed. I'm talking about the kind of practical advice that doctors wouldn't really know about. The doctor can tell you what medication to take, but only a peer with the same issue can tell you when is the best time to get your refill because there won't be a long line at the clinic at that time of day, and which bus is the one you want to take because it has far fewer stops, so you'll get there quicker. That kind of peer support provides people with a friend with a similar condition, living in the same community. We have been able to support those peer-to-peer relationships, which are generating better health outcomes, through our flexible services.

iTunes gift cards? Bicycles? Yoga studio memberships? A friend with the same medical condition who can tell you which bus to take and what hour of the day will save you the most time when you get your refill? In the traditional healthcare model, there's simply no way to pay for these types of goods and services. There's also no place for the imagination of healthcare providers (and their patients) to sprout ideas that could then be turned into programs to get better healthcare outcomes while driving down the cost of care.

The concept of *flexible services* is not a panacea. It's not as though we could just take a bunch of money and throw it at every healthcare problem under the sun and get better outcomes. So far, we have had great success, both in creating a methodology for spending these dollars with deep input from our healthcare provider communities, and in terms of the results we have achieved. Flexible services are a critical part of the solution when it comes to improving healthcare outcomes, not just in Yamhill County, or even in the state of Oregon, but everywhere in the nation.

CHAPTER 12:

CAN THIS WORK EVERYWHERE ELSE?

The issues we have faced in Yamhill County, plus or minus, are the issues that all communities across the country face every day. Healthcare spending is on the rise. Patients and healthcare providers alike are frustrated because they aren't getting great results. There is an intense desire for the situation to improve. Insurance companies are increasing their sway. There is a lack of communication among the various types of healthcare providers in any given community: hospitals, doctors, dentists, social workers, psychologists, addictions counselors, and so on. And there is a burgeoning caseload of Medicaid patients, thanks to the Affordable Care Act.

Obviously, what we're doing in Yamhill County, and in Oregon in general, would have to be modified to meet the specific needs of every community. At the same time, what we're doing here could work just about anywhere.

Urban areas have their own challenges, given the larger number of people packed into a smaller geographic locations. And yet, Oregon has urban CCOs that are doing similar work to what we've seen in Yamhill County. In larger cities like Chicago, each ward could be its own CCO. It just depends on how you define community and whether you can put the right people into leadership positions. Can it work anywhere? It can certainly improve things anywhere, that's for sure.

If you're concerned that this might not work in your community because a meaningful percentage of your patients are of cultural or ethnic diversity, remember that in Yamhill County, 16 percent of our patients are Hispanic. We consciously made our leadership bilingual and inclusive. Things don't have to be one-size-fits-all. That's the good news.

So how do you begin? Go to the providers in your community—the doctors, the nurses, the behaviorists, the dentists, and so on. Tell them you want them to be involved in this process and take part in this leadership. They probably haven't had that choice or opportunity in the past.

Trust the community to self-organize. All you must do is provide the basic structure and then they can decide how exactly the whole thing will work. Reach out to hospitals, government officials, Head Start folks, and so on. The greater the outreach at the beginning of the process, the more likely you'll get buy-in from the people you need on board.

Keep in mind that you cannot force doctors to do what's best for them any more easily than you can "force" patients to comply with your prescriptions and directives. It's not about telling people they must be a part of it; it's about asking people.

Here, providers saw the value of the whole thing, so they came together and got it done.

Our three community health workers are all bilingual and bicultural, which was intentional, so that we could address our Hispanic population. The leadership doesn't necessarily have to be bicultural or bilingual, but the people who serve the community should be.

Another challenge in many communities is that the hospital systems are one of the biggest players in town. Sometimes, they're even bigger than local government, because they are often the largest employer in an area and they have the biggest budgets, the most revenue, and the highest expenses. They may not be politically involved in a traditional sense, like operating on a county board or helping to set legislative policies. Yet, in a model like a CCO, hospitals can be something like the eight-hundred-pound gorilla in the room.

In Yamhill, we have been fortunate to have two hospital systems that essentially balance one another. One is a large, independent hospital that is owned by an out-of-state medical corporation. The smaller one is part of a larger regional system known as the Providence Health System.

If you're going to go down the path of developing a CCO, I cannot stress how important it is for the hospitals and other frontline providers to be involved. These are the folks who see the problems most extensively, deal with the patients, and take home the headaches and the heartaches at the end of the day. These are the hospitals, the individual family practice doctors, and other primary care providers.

In the latter case, it might just be the doctor, a nurse in his office, and his teenage daughter working the front desk. In a CCO, the doctor's voice might carry more weight than the

CEO of a multimillion-dollar hospital, because he's out there actually seeing people and recognizing the issues. He's also the one who must implement any decisions and find a way to get paid at the end of the day. So, don't let the fact that there are larger stakeholders of any kind dissuade you from trying to start something like this. At the same time, involve them from the start, because their voices matter.

If you want to create your own CCO, first see if there is some existing structure within which you could work. As I've described throughout the book, we had a mandate from the state of Oregon to create this kind of change. Thus, we had rules and requirements about what needed to go into a CCO. In our case, the legislation specified that it had to have a board of directors, including at least one physician in active practice, at least one representative from local county government and at least one behavioral health provider. That set of rules gave us a basic framework with which to start. Perhaps there is an existing set of legislative rules regarding healthcare in your state, or a stakeholder who wants to find a new way to deliver care. Perhaps it's an insurance company desirous of forming an ACO or developing a new way of delivering more coordinated care in a community. If there's a simple framework out there already, consider using it.

If there is no such framework, that's fine, too. You can still come together and use some of the elements that we have used, as appropriate for your community. Just make sure that you are engaging a diverse group of stakeholders from across the community, including those who are involved in influencing the "determinants of health"—the things we've discussed that happen outside the doctor's office.

In other words, you want not just medical care and behavioral healthcare folks, but also individuals who represent the socioeconomic interests in your community, like the head of a local Head Start program or people involved in transportation, housing, or job skills. Perhaps you can involve someone from the local Department of Public Health. The broader the representation of community stakeholders, the more likely that you're going to succeed. I was a big proponent of including leaders from the various sectors of the community that addressed the so-called social determinants of health.

In our model, the board of directors acts as the voice of the payer, because they're the ones making decisions about rates and what kinds of programs get funded. You need to make sure you have a board of balanced stakeholders.

The board also needs to be informed by the providers delivering care of the identity of the patients receiving it. We do so by having a Clinical Advisory Panel (CAP) composed of different providers from around the community. They help set different clinical policies and help to develop transformative programs to deliver healthcare in new and different ways.

We also have our Community Advisory Council (CAC), where the members (the patients) or their family members can give input. It's really a three-legged stool: the providers, the payers, and the patients. When all three are represented, the whole thing balances.

Then you build the organization the way you would any other. We started first by developing our mission, vision, and a set of guiding principles. This was largely accomplished by the CAC and the community members the organization serves. Then we focused on metrics: How will we be measured for the sorts of things we want to provide? Then, how do we meet those metrics and stay within our budget while living within the spirit of our mission, vision, and guiding principles?

Once we had worked out the basics around these issues, we had to provide to the state of Oregon, in clear detail, the exact nature of our plan for transforming healthcare. We addressed eight elements in our formally titled "Transformation Plan." Here are some of the key ones:

- Improving health information technology in our community
- Getting different providers to talk to each other, not only on the phone or in meetings, but also electronically through EMRs and other platforms
- Increasing the number of our members enrolled in patient-centered primary care homes or so-called "super clinics"
- Paying for *value* of healthcare delivery and not just *volume*
- Addressing diversity, ensuring cultural competence, language training, and sensitivity to issues affecting different ethnicities

It's an extremely valuable and necessary exercise to create a plan like this, because then you end up with a blueprint that everyone can accept.

Next, we had to align that eight-point transformation plan with our metrics, to make sure that our efforts would produce legitimate outcomes that could be tracked by external parties, with payments attached to it. Once you've got this in place, you can go to a health insurer and say, "We want to do this for the community. Will you contract with us? Can we manage your population of members living in our community with this health plan?"

It might seem absurd or unworkable at first, but this approach really puts the control of governing healthcare resources into the hands of people who live in the community and who appreciate those services, the individuals who are invested in seeing those outcomes. These are the folks getting paid for doing the work or receiving the care.

To put it simply, this works. This model is an opportunity to move beyond what typically happens when an outside third-party payer—one that just wants to contract with doctors and pay for their services on a one-off basis—is simply repeating the same old song and dance. In a typical arrangement, the providers are trying to negotiate for a higher rate every year, and the payers are trying to increase rates on their members. The members, of course, are unsatisfied with the diminishing scope of the services they receive. In our model, we've been able to provide an alternative to that unsatisfying and unrewarding exercise.

We now have a platform that works for Medicaid members. Yamhill could now potentially go and work with commercial payers and offer its whole network of services to commercially insured members so that they could take advantage of all the great services we offer, like our Persistent Pain Program.

Unfortunately, those with commercial insurance in Yamhill County do not have access to all these great services; at least, they don't right now. Our next step could be to go to commercial insurers and contract with them to bear the risk for the lives they must cover, so that we can offer them the services we have developed for Medicaid.

Then we can also address the dilemma that many providers face: What percentage of their panel of patients should be Medicaid patients? Classically, Medicaid pays only about half of what commercial insurance pays, so many providers will limit their percentage of Medicaid patients to 10 to 20 percent. With our model, if we can get other payers on board, we could offer a single rate to the providers who contract with us and pay them the same for all the patients they see, whether they are Medicaid patients or commercially insured patients.

We could then tell providers, "We'll pay you the same amount for either Medicaid patients or commercially insured patients. We will measure your performance with both groups by the same set of metrics. You can be paid based on meeting those metrics, so that you can develop programs, hire staff, and implement different resources to help you meet those performance criteria. These are resources that can then be applied across your whole patient population; you would not be offering these services only to Medicaid patients."

Thus, you've got a community where everyone has access to the same level of care, which is, quite frankly, how things should be.

Does this sound like a healthcare utopia? Not exactly. We still have our challenges, and we are still inventing and reinventing ourselves on the fly. The good news is that, with each passing year, our CCO here in Yamhill County and the CCO networks across the state of Oregon are getting stronger, more efficient, and more effective. CCOs are delivering better and better results to the people who need it most.

It is my fervent wish that you see something in our model that you can apply to your community, as well. I would love to hear how things work out for you in that regard. And if you have any desire to come visit us in Oregon and see how we do things, we welcome you!

AFTERWORD

Since completing the writing of this book, Donald Trump has been elected President and serious questions exist as to the future of Obamacare. The relevant question to this book is, will all the work I described potentially vanish if the ACA is done away with ? The answer is mixed, in some ways yes and in others no.

Oregon recently was awarded a new waiver from CMS in January 2017 to continue the coordinated care model and its CCOs for another five years. With that, the structure of the CCO's, the metrics, the novel programs, and the CCO's themselves are able to remain in place. What could possibly be at stake are the approximately 400,000 Oregonians who gained coverage under the expansion of Medicaid in Oregon with Obamacare. If the Medicaid expansion is rolled back, these individuals could loss Medicaid benefits and their enrollment in CCO's. It is unclear what the impact this would have on CCOs and local communities.

I will say, the CCO structure is successful no matter what side of the political aisle you view it from and would go a long way to inform any type of new national healthcare reform efforts. The model has kept healthcare spending under 3.4% growth per year of five years straight. It is an accountable system to the federal government, providers and patients with its set of performance metrics. Local communities are given control of their healthcare resources along with the ability to bear financial risk and risk for clinical outcomes. Finally, the model fosters innovation which builds on relationships and organizational development without needing protracted research and spending.

I invite political and policy leaders to look at the results of Oregon's coordinated care model to see how it can serve as a blueprint or essential element of future national healthcare reforms. Coordinated care works for Oregon and can work for all communities in the United States.

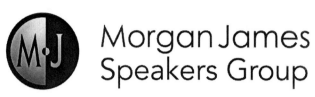

Morgan James
Speakers Group

We connect Morgan James published authors with live and online events and audiences whom will benefit from their expertise.

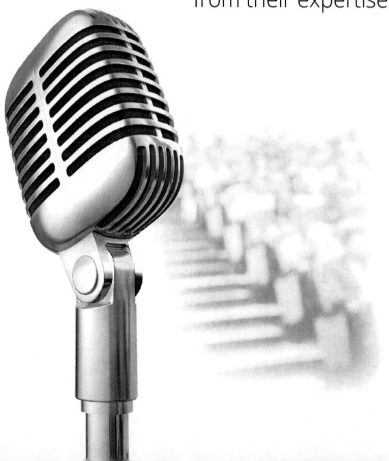

CPSIA information can be obtained
at www.ICGtesting.com
Printed in the USA
LVOW12*0533261017
553802LV00003BA/26/P

9 781683 502999